Multiple Choice Questions for the MRCPsych Part I

Examination

The Multiple Choice Question in Psychiatry Series

Multiple Choice Questions for the MRCPsych Part I

Examination

E. Jane Marshall, MRCPI, MRCPsych
Consultant Psychiatrist and Senior Lecturer, Maudsley Hospital, Denmark Hill, London

Foreword by

Professor David Goldberg
Professor of Psychiatry, Institute of Psychiatry, London

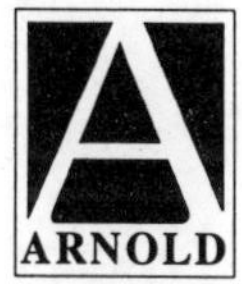

A member of the Hodder Headline Group
LONDON • NEW YORK • NEW DELHI

First published in Great Britain in 1995 by Butterworth Heinemann.

This impression published in 2002 by
Arnold, a member of the Hodder Headline Group,
338 Euston Road, London NW1 3BH

http://www.arnoldpublishers.com

Co-published in the USA by
Oxford University Press Inc.,
198 Madison Avenue, New York, NY10016
Oxford is a registered trademark of Oxford University Press

British Library Cataloguing in Publication Data
A catalogue record for this book is available from the British Library

Library of Congress Cataloging-in-Publication Data
A catalog record for this book is available from the Library of Congress

ISBN 0 7506 1871 X

3 4 5 6 7 8 9 10

Printed and bound in India by Replika Press Pvt Ltd., 100% EOU,
Delhi-110 040

Contents

Foreword to series

As the authors rightly say in Chapter 4, for most candidates examinations are an ordeal – disruptive, onerous, worrying and tedious. Nothing can be done to remove the anxiety completely, to banish the burden, or to eliminate the tedium. However, in so far as anything can lighten the candidate's burden or to replace terror with hope, these books are it.

When the College was first set up, the old Royal Medico-Psychological Association sought to model itself on the College of Physicians of London, which at that time made rather little effort to maintain standards of training posts, but expended much effort on devising a punitive examination with a very high failure rate. A deputation of dissidents from the Maudsley protested about these plans, and demanded that the new College should have a major concern with ensuring that candidates for the future examination received a proper clinical training. Two members of this deputation were later to become President of the College and Chief Examiner, and I think that all the others have served the College as Examiners.

The College has a proud record in having ensured that training schemes were set up in such a way that young psychiatrists receive a balanced training, and that consultants take their teaching responsibilities seriously. Unlike most other colleges, ours has a nationwide system of clinical tutors charged with specific responsibilities towards trainees. This being so, one cannot complain if the College also sets a searching professional examination for its potential members.

In the years since the College was set up there have been enormous advances in our understanding of both basic and clinical neuroscience, and less dramatic but still substantial advances in knowledge in social psychiatry. The most demanding test of this knowledge is embodied in the three multiple choice question (MCQ) examinations set by the College.

These books do three things well: they acquaint the candidate with examples of up-to-date test material across the entire range of the examination; they increase the candidate's knowledge by giving informative answers accompanied by references to original papers dealing with the test materials, and they shamelessly teach candidates the tricks of the trade to ensure that they get the highest possible mark for the level of knowledge that they in fact possess by the time the examination comes round.

In reading through the test material that makes up the bulk of these three volumes I have been impressed by how much I learned myself. I had thought that I had kept up with my reading since the time when I completed my own examinations – but often when I strayed from my own areas of special interest I found that I was learning new material by attempting the test material and then checking my responses against the helpful notes that follow on the next page.

Those who work their way through this book are likely to emerge as better-informed psychiatrists. If they have to sit the MCQ examination, they will undoubtedly obtain a much higher score than before. It seems almost unfair – but there is nothing improper about it.

Professor David Goldberg
Professor of Psychiatry, Institute of Psychiatry

Preface

The *Multiple Choice Questions in Psychiatry* series comprises three volumes – one for each of the three MCQ papers in the MRCPsych examination. This volume is designed to prepare candidates for the MRCPsych Part I multiple choice examination paper. The other two volumes are for the MRCPsych Part II Clinical Topics paper and the MRCPsych Part II Sciences basic to psychiatry paper. Section I of each book has been written jointly by the series' authors and tailored to the particular examination being addressed.

Multiple choice examinations are an objective method of assessing candidates, but are as much a test of MCQ technique as they are of knowledge. Candidates wishing to pass the MRCPsych Part I examination should approach their revision with this in mind. This MCQ book is not merely a collection of practice questions; it aims to teach as much as to test. Questions relevant to the syllabus have been devised and are based on standard textbooks, key papers from the leading psychiatric journals and papers cited in the Reading List of the Royal College of Psychiatrists. Explanations, notes and references to further reading have been added to most of the answers. A subject index has been included to assist candidates revise specific topics.

Each question has been scrutinized by examination candidates and other psychiatrists at the Maudsley Hospital and rated for factual accuracy, ambiguity, relevance, difficulty and so forth. As a result, many question items were rejected, leaving, we hope, three collections of question papers of a standard as close as possible to that required in the examination. Any errors remaining in this volume are entirely mine.

The first section of the book aims to help candidates to prepare for the MCQ papers by reviewing first, the nature and regulations of the exam; second, the principles underlying the setting of MCQs; and third, revision/examination technique. Candidates are strongly recommended to read this section before proceeding to the papers.

The questions were constructed at a time coinciding with the arrival of the 10th edition of the *International Classification of Diseases* (*ICD-*

10; World Health Organization, 1992) and the 4th edition of the *Diagnostic and Statistical Manual* of the American Psychiatric Association (*DSM–IV*; American Psychiatric Association, 1994). Accordingly, these have been adopted.

I am very grateful to all those who assessed the questions, particularly Dr Kathryn Abel, Dr Katherine Aitchison, Dr Dominic Ffytche, Dr Rafia Ghubash, Dr Nick Goddard, Dr Sonia Johnson, Dr Chris McEvedy, Dr Oscar Meehan, Dr Edward Petch, Dr Emma Staples, Dr Mark Taylor and Dr Cleo van Velsen and many others. I should like to thank Mrs Sandi Sari for secretarial assistance.

Mr Michael Jackson initiated the idea for this project and provided encouragement as it developed.

E. Jane Marshall
Maudsley Hospital, London

Section I

1

How to use this book

> We say. Loke yer thou lepe, whose literall sence is, doo nothinge sodenly or without avisement. *W. Tyndale (1528)*

This book, like its sister volumes in the *Multiple Choice Questions in Psychiatry* series, has been prepared with the following aims in mind:

1. To provide instruction on the principles and intentions behind the setting of MCQs in the hope that you will derive information that will be of assistance in answering this form of question.
2. To provide advice and guidance on the nature of the MRCPsych Part I examination and on aspects of the regulations.
3. To equip you with the expertise and skills with which to answer MCQs.
4. To supply you with detailed advice on how to organize and carry out your revision.
5. To improve your final preparation for the examination, particularly on how to conduct yourself before the examination begins and to improve the way you take the examination.
6. To provide practice examination papers that will enable you to rehearse your technique, assess your knowledge and acquire new knowledge.

This first section contains important preparatory chapters and it is strongly recommended that these are studied carefully before the examination papers are attempted – Tyndale's words remain relevant over four centuries later! Chapter 2 contains an outline of the nature of the MRCPsych Part I examination, and the syllabus on which the MCQ paper is based. The third chapter is designed to better your understanding of MCQs – the principles used in their construction and the implications of certain terms that they commonly contain. The fourth chapter considers how to revise for the examination, and discusses how to take the examination. Section I concludes with an important résumé of the rules and principles that you should use both to prepare for the examination and to sit it.

In Section II the practice MCQ questions are arranged into five mock examination papers. It is strongly recommended that you use the response sheets and do each of these practice papers under examination conditions. Having read the section on how to pass the examination you will wish to rehearse different approaches to doing the questions, noting the advantages of each.

Each question is followed by an answer and a reference to further reading. I have endeavoured to compose the questions from the reference material based on the recommended reading lists published by the Royal College of Psychiatrists, the more authoritative textbooks, and important review articles and papers from psychiatric journals.

The composition of the practice examination papers reflects the syllabus published in the regulations and the blend of topics used in the 25 MCQs of the sample paper published by the Royal College of Psychiatrists.

Recent candidates report that the questions in this series are pitched at about the correct level. The level of difficulty of a given question is partly subjective; candidates will cite different questions as being easy or difficult.

It may be felt that a few questions are a little obscure – relevance was one criterion on which the questions were rated by a panel of assessors, yet, as it transpired, the only criterion on which the panel regularly disagreed. The author's approach to this matter has been to include information that will add to a candidate's general psychiatric education even if it may not necessarily appear to be of immediate relevance to the MCQ section of the examination – such questions are few, however.

Each entry in the reference section is cross-referenced to the question(s) for which it has been a source. This will allow you to check your knowledge on aspects of this reference, though do remember that most of these references contain a great detail of additional information that is not tested in the MCQ.

2

The MRCPsych Part I examination

Information

General information and regulations for the MRCPsych examinations are published by the Royal College of Psychiatrists. Since these are subject to regular amendment, the candidate is strongly advised to write to the College for the most current regulations. Ensure that you know the closing dates for completed applications well in advance. Many candidates apply in a last-minute rush and inevitably some actually miss the date. Application forms are available on written request to the Examinations Department.

The address of the Royal College of Psychiatrists is:

The Royal College of Psychiatrists
17 Belgrave Square
London
SW1X 8PG

Entry requirements for the MRCPsych Part I

Entry requirements are detailed in *General Information and Regulations for the MRCPsych Examinations*, published by the Royal College of Psychiatrists (1994).

In general, candidates must have completed 12 months of full-time (or equivalent part-time) approved psychiatric training for the Part I examination. They must also satisfy the College's registration and sponsorship requirements.

Approved psychiatric training

The candidate should have had practical clinical experience in psychiatry in a training post approved by the Royal College of Psychiatrists and should also have attended an appropriate academic course. Twelve months of adult general psychiatry or 6 months each of adult general psychiatry and psychiatry of old age will fulfil the requirements. The minimum duration of any one appointment must be not less than 6 months.

In the UK and the Republic of Ireland training as a senior house officer or a registrar is accepted. Training in a staff-grade post which has been approved by the Dean for the MRCPsych examinations is also accepted. Requirements for overseas candidates are set out in detail in the document. Ensure that you understand the entry requirements at the beginning of your training, not when you are about to apply to sit the examination.

Exemptions

Holders of the following recognized overseas qualifications are exempt from the MRCPsych Part I:

1. Australia and New Zealand: FRANZCP.
2. Canada: FRCP (Psych) Canada.
3. USA: American Board Examination in Psychiatry.

Registration

Candidates training in the UK should normally be registered with the General Medical Council. Candidates training in the Republic of Ireland should normally be registered with the Irish Medical Council. Full details regarding candidates who are not registered as above are set out in the *General Information and Regulations for the MRCPsych Examinations* (Royal College of Psychiatrists, 1994).

Sponsorship

At each attempt candidates should be supported by statements from two consultants (sponsors) – one from the candidate's psychiatric tutor and the other from a consultant with whom the candidate has worked for at least 6 months preceding the date of application. Sponsors are asked to confirm that the candidate has had satisfactory training in a range of stated areas. Make sure that you identify your sponsors in good time.

Format of the examination

The Part I examination is an examination in basic clinical psychiatry. Knowledge of the subject and practical skills are accorded equal importance. The examination consists of:

1. One multiple choice paper (1 hour 30 minutes, 50 questions).
2. One clinical examination (1 hour 30 minutes).

Content of the multiple choice paper

Basic psychopathology: descriptive and explanatory

1. A basic knowledge of the phenomenology of psychiatry and the ways in which symptoms and signs are expressed and experienced.
2. An awareness of the internal (personality and developmental) and external (environmental) influences which can cause and shape these phenomena.
3. An understanding of the principles underlying the classification of the phenomena into syndromes.

Methods of clinical assessment in psychiatry
The candidate should understand the principles underlying the clinical methods of psychiatry – the establishing of a satisfactory working relationship with the patient, the eliciting of a satisfactory psychiatric history, the procedures for examining the patient's mental state and related abnormalities on physical examination, and the integrating of this information in clinical assessment with recognition of the need for further examination and/or investigations.

Basic clinical psychopharmacology
This covers the basic principles of pharmacokinetics and drug action in relation to the main groups of drugs used in psychiatry – anxiolytics, antidepressives, antipsychotics, sedatives/hypnotics, lithium and anticonvulsants.

Neuroanatomy, neurophysiology and neuropathology

Neuroanatomy: Knowledge of the brain and spinal cord and peripheral nervous system as the basis of the neurological examination and diagnosis.

Neurophysiology: Physiology of the motor and sensory systems and the autonomic nervous system.

Neuropathology: Principal neuropathological changes in degenerative disorders, cerebrovascular disorders and other conditions which may be referred to the psychiatrist.

How this relates to the MCQ paper can be assessed by looking at the sample paper published by the College. However, it should be noted that

Table 1

Clinical topic	*Number of questions*
Descriptive psychopathology	30
Dynamic psychopathology	6
Basic clinical psychopharmacology	8
Neuroanatomy, neurophysiology and neuropathology	6
Total	50

this paper is only an example and the balance of topics chosen for each examination could vary considerably. Nevertheless, analysis of the 25 questions in the specimen paper implies that a 50-question paper would have a breakdown of topics as given in Table 1.

Pass mark

To be successful, candidates must pass the clinical examination and achieve a standard in the MCQ paper which is acceptable to the Examinations Subcommittee. There is no single pass mark for the MCQ papers and candidates are advised to score as highly as possible (Morgan and Hill, 1991).

Number of attempts and the time allowed for attempts

From Spring 1994 candidates are allowed a maximum of four attempts at the MRCPsych Part I examination over a period of 4 years of full-time or equivalent part-time approved psychiatric training.

Feedback to candidates who have not succeeded

Unsuccessful candidates can write to the Chief Examiner before the closing date, for feedback. Feedback is only given on the section in which they have failed. It is usually comprehensive and helpful, highlighting in a general manner those areas in which there are deficiencies.

Summary

1. Current examination regulations are available through a written application to the Examination Department of the Royal College of Psychiatrists.
2. The entry requirements should be studied early in your training, not just before you apply.
3. Identify your potential sponsors and understand their role.
4. Ensure you understand how you are going to be examined. Orient your learning to this.
5. Note carefully the breadth of the syllabus and ensure that your training and revision cover as much of this as is possible.
6. There is no pass mark in the MCQ papers. Aim to score as highly as you can.

3

The multiple choice question

It is of considerable advantage when preparing for an MCQ examination to understand how MCQs are constructed. Of the many sources available for this purpose, the account by Anderson, on which much of the following advice is based, remains the most authoritative and useful (Anderson, 1976).

Why use MCQs at all?

The MCQ format grew out of a need to have an objective method to assess and rank candidates and has been the subject of debate by John Anderson and Sir George Pickering (Anderson, 1979, 1981; Pickering, 1979).

Unlike essays and orals, the well-constructed MCQ examination paper excludes the subjective bias of examiners and ensures all candidates are examined on the same material. Candidates are discouraged from hasty guessing by the adoption of negative marking – the deduction of a mark for an incorrect response. This is a stratagem that also simplifies the process of discriminating between candidates.

It should be emphasized that the well-constructed MCQ paper is an ideal to which examination authors aspire but often fail to achieve since there are many pitfalls; the experience of sitting on examination committees that review questions quickly shows that it is not at all uncommon for questions to advance into an examination paper still imperfect in one respect or another. Furthermore, not all knowledge areas in psychiatry lend themselves to examination by MCQ (Strauss *et al.*, 1982).

What principles do examiners follow when constructing MCQs and can knowledge of these principles be of assistance to you?

Examiners seek to produce well-constructed questions in plain English that follow the syllabus and discriminate adequately between candidates of varying ability. There are certain rules or principles and, in some circumstances, as we shall see, if you are knowledgeable about the setting of MCQs you can use stylistic errors and grammatical clues to your advantage.

What are the various components of MCQ questions called?

There is a set of precise terms that are used to describe the component parts of the MCQ and it is well worth getting to know them. These are given in Table 2.

Table 2 Definitions of terms used to describe aspects of the MCQ

Term	*Definition*
True	One of the three recognized responses to a question. Such a response may be correct or incorrect; true and correct are not synonymous
False	One of the three recognized responses to a question. Such a response may be correct or incorrect; false and incorrect are not synonymous
Don't know	One of the three recognized responses to a question. No marks are awarded or deducted for using this response
Stem	The introductory statement which, together with an option, forms one of the five component questions of an MCQ
Option	The stem is followed by five options, labelled A to E. Each option (sometimes called a *completion*) will, in combination with the stem, form a discrete question, known as an item. Each of the five items in a given MCQ is independent of the other four.
Item	The stem and option together form an item. In College examinations a given MCQ will contain five component items
Distractor	An item for which the correct response is *false*

Modified from Anderson (1976).

Use of English

MCQs should employ plain English that is precise and to the point. Unfortunately, where this is not achieved, you may face ambiguity or, where English is not your first language, actual disadvantage.

Breadth and depth of the questions

The examination should be set to reflect the syllabus and the questions pitched at an appropriate level of difficulty. From the examiners' point of view, if the questions are too easy, the scores will not discriminate between candidates of varying calibre. If you have an especially advanced knowledge of a particular topic, you should not overread the question; that is, you should assume the examiners are setting it at the level of a good to advanced clinician, not that of an advanced research worker. Many candidates create ambiguity in their minds in this way, and if you find this happening, you need to muse on what the examiners' intention was.

Some guidance on the intended level in Royal College examinations can be gauged from the original sample question paper provided by the college, though recent questions are substantially harder than these. At the level of specialist medical examinations, examiners are rarely devious and should be trusted.

Certain words and phrases crop up regularly in MCQs – should they be interpreted in a particular way?

Some words and phrases (Table 3) do have a generally accepted usage and therefore you must be entirely familiar with them. Question practice will help considerably. Vigilance is required and if there is plenty of time left at the end, double-check your interpretation of any question item containing these words and phrases.

Negatives require a special mention. Examiners usually avoid them, but inevitably they creep in, often when there is a need to make the correct response to an item a little less obvious. Approach negatives, especially double-negatives, with caution and, again, you might check you have interpreted them correctly if there is time at the end of the examination.

The word 'may' still appears in the wording of MCQs, despite criticism of its use (Bisson, 1991). Essentially the word 'may' implies a possibility, however remote, and thus True is likely to be the correct

Table 3 Definitions of words widely used in the stems and options of MCQ questions

Word	*Definition*
Characteristic	A word that has a specific meaning – a characteristic feature is a feature that would be expected to occur for the diagnosis to be made, and where absent would lead to some doubt about the diagnosis
Commonly	A term that should be taken to mean an event that occurs more than 50% of the time
Pathognomonic	A pathognomonic feature implies the feature being referred to occurs in the disease or disorder named only, and in no other
Recognized	A recognized feature is a feature of a disorder that has been reported and which a candidate would reasonably be expected to know of. Characteristic features are always recognized but the reverse may not be the case
Special	A term generally used in the same way as pathognomonic
Typical	A term that should be taken as a synonym for characteristic

Modified from Anderson (1976).

answer, though not always. Absolute words such as 'always' and 'never' are usually avoided by examiners as the correct response is so rarely anything but False. If you come across these you will usually be correct to guess False; those few where True really is the correct answer will hopefully be apparent to you!

Examiners seek to avoid phrases such as 'has been associated with' but they are still to be found. The implied meaning is 'has been known to be described in conjunction with at some time or other' and candidates should recognize this grammatical clue, which will rarely be False.

Slade and Dewey (1983) have studied the role of grammatical clues in MCQ examinations and reach interesting conclusions.

By scrutinizing the sample paper of the old Preliminary Test of the Royal College of Psychiatrists, a list of 34 words and phrases was produced which it was felt contained grammatical features that tended to discriminate between True and False response items (Table 4).

The authors looked to see if these grammatical clues could be applied to MCQs other than those from which they were derived. They could, and with some considerable benefit. It was found that 18% of a random sample of 600 question items in a widely used MCQ book could be responded to from grammatical clues alone, and almost four-fifths of these (80 out of 107) would have been answered correctly. Thus, a

Table 4 Positive and negative key words and phrases

True responses	*False responses*
May	Always
May be	Necessarily
Can be	Is necessarily
Can appear	Characteristically
Tend(s)	Typically
Contribute to	All
Is of benefit	First
Of value	Appropriate
Useful	Same as
Suggest(s)	The fact that
Is possible	Do(es) not
Encourages	Requires
Are (is) often	No value
Are (is) frequently	Are free from
Have (has) been	Is complete
Usually	Very useful
	Is important
	Essential

From Slade and Dewey (1983), with permission.
Note: this table is included to illustrate the research discussed in the text; it should not be assumed that these words can be used in the examination to predict what the correct response might be.

candidate could get a positive score of 53 (80 minus 27) without using any factual knowledge – almost 9% of the question items. They went on to show that subjects do obtain higher scores on items that contain grammatical clues, particularly where they are contained in the option.

As in practice it is hard to set MCQ papers free from grammatical clues, it would seem that the candidate who is aware of these clues, and uses this knowledge *with care*, could potentially raise the score he or she has derived from factual knowledge alone – potentially taking the score over the threshold of a pass.

Precision with terms

Examiners seek to set clear questions, but imprecision can slip in unnoticed. For example, the term schizophrenia may be used without qualification as to what subtype, if any, is being referred to. Rather than leave the question out, once again you should trust that the examiner is not being devious.

Eponymous names, while not necessarily unfair, are best qualified in brackets; where not, the examiner may often be relied upon to have left a clue to the disorder in the options supplied. Drug doses or percentages may be stated in a way that implies that a figure differing by a small amount would be wrong. You may realize such precision is wrong and be tempted to use the response 'Don't know' because of the ambiguity created. It is better, however, just to accept the examiner's slip and assume the figure to be correct if it is in the right area. You should feel justifiably aggrieved if only the trade name of a drug is given – in practice, however, this is most unlikely to occur.

The relationship between items

In the multiple True/False variety of questions favoured to date by the Royal College of Psychiatrists, each item should be independent and not interrelated. If you are unsure of the answer to an item, check to ensure this rule has been followed – while it is uncommon, occasionally items will be found to be interdependent. Questions, as well as items, should be independent. Sometimes you may find hints to the answer of an item in another question.

Scrambling

Researchers have spotted a tendency for questions to be ordered with one or two True items followed by a series of distractors. Examiners will often therefore mix up or scramble the items so that there is no such tendency. Just occasionally unscrambled questions appear with a strong tendency for the initial item to be True. Recognition of this may be of assistance in constructing an informed guess, though it is potentially very hazardous to guess on this basis alone.

Summary

1. There is a generally accepted set of principles governing the setting of MCQ questions. It is advantageous to understand these rules.
2. Take the time to learn the definition of terms such as item, distractor and stem.
3. Avoid overreading the difficulty of questions – become familiar with the general standard required by your examiners.
4. Learn the meaning of terms such as characteristic, typical and recognized.

5. Familiarize yourself with the correct interpretation of words and phrases that may provide grammatical clues.
6. Care is required not only in interpreting terms that have been used with excessive precision but also with those that are used imprecisely.
7. Interrelated items in a question, while uncommon, may provide clues to the correct response.

4

Passing the examination

Preparation

When to start your revision?

You will have started to read and learn about psychiatry the day you entered the discipline, if not sooner. Before you enter the period of final revision for the Part I, it is of great advantage to have several months of steady work behind you. Such work should include regular reading of journals such as the *British Journal of Psychiatry*, and relevant features in the *British Medical Journal* and other publications. Hopefully you will have kept up with your background reading, particularly by reading up unfamiliar topics *as they arose* (this takes the mystique out of clinical topics and confidence rapidly accrues). When reading, it may be of value to bear in mind how the more factual material might be adapted for examination in an MCQ (Smyth, 1991).

Individuals will vary in the time they give to their revision. Six months seems about right for most – any longer and you may find it hard to sustain your interest, any less and the task may be more of a struggle. It is beneficial to try to be ready 2 weeks before the exam – in practice this will be liable to slip to a week or less.

What books to use?

Use a few core texts but know them well. The books listed in Table 5 are good *core* reference texts for the MRCPsych Part I. Avoid the tendency to consult too many sources, with the risk of ending up with a bewildering collection of barely used books. There can be little doubt that if those listed are systematically studied then you will be left with few gaps, especially if one or two journals are regularly read. The *ICD* and *DSM* manuals are perhaps surprising inclusions – no apology is made, for they are both succinct and precise compilations of the

Table 5 Suggested core texts and journals required for passing the MCQ Clinical Topics section of the MRCPsych Part I examination

A textbook of psychiatry (e.g. the *Oxford Textbook of Psychiatry*; the *Companion to Psychiatric Studies*). (*Reading one text alone will not suffice; it will need to be supplemented with additional focused reading, particularly in the areas outlined below*)
A guide to drug treatments (e.g. *British National Formulary* – don't overlook the wealth of information here; Silverstone and Turner, 1988)
A guide to history-taking (e.g. 'the orange book', Institute of Psychiatry, 1987)
A guide to phenomenology (e.g. Kräupl-Taylor, 1979; Fish (Hamilton, 1985); Sims, 1988)
The *ICD-10* and *DSM–IV* manuals (succinct and authoritative clarity which is hard to find elsewhere)
Practice MCQ examination books
British Journal of Psychiatry; *Psychiatric Bulletin (Royal College of Psychiatrists)*; *Psychological Medicine*; *British Medical Journal* (editorials especially); *Current Opinion in Psychiatry*; *International Review of Psychiatry*; *British Journal of Hospital Medicine*

recognized psychiatric disorders and are invaluable for understanding nosology and classification. When you are familiar with these, difficulty with differential diagnosis and formulations will be long past. Many questions produced in this book are from the books and journals listed.

How to get organized?

Careful attention to the organization of your revision will be of huge value to you. For each aspect of the Part I examination you should devise a revision strategy. It will become immediately apparent that there is a lot to do. It is important to set targets or time will fritter away in inefficient study. Balance is required – for example, it will be of little help to know phenomenology inside out, if the rest of the syllabus is neglected. You may have to compromise on your initial objectives – corners will have to be cut and material left out.

As useful background, many candidates find it advantageous to write a summary of a clinical text or two, chapter by chapter in condensed note form so as to form concise, background reference notes which are readily memorized. A similar approach can be taken to learning other key material.

It is ideal to approach the various sections of the examination in parallel. Enterprising candidates will rally more senior colleagues to give practice in the oral sections of the examination, preferably at regular times each week.

What to do for the MCQ paper?

As mentioned above, the preparation for this MCQ paper should be integrated into your total revision programme. Much of the factual knowledge will accumulate from the reading that you have undertaken. After first devoting time to studying MCQ question technique, you should get lots of practice in doing questions. Your adeptness at doing MCQs will increase, as will your factual base, especially if you use MCQs that are supplied with explanatory answers and references. You should ideally make brief notes of new pieces of information. Arrange these under the main clinical headings in the syllabus, allowing a sheet of paper for each heading. It is especially advantageous for you to sit practice examinations such as those contained in this book. As you do this, assess your technique as well as your factual knowledge. Technique is considered in detail below.

How to keep going?

For some candidates, examinations are no problem; for many, if not most, they are an ordeal – disruptive, onerous, worrying and tedious. There is no antidote, though it can help if you analyse how you are bearing up. First, you can ease your worry by remembering successes in past examination hurdles that have been overcome – think positively!

Second, you may recall from your reading that, according to the Yerkes-Dodson law, a moderate degree of anxiety seems to promote performance; indeed, remember your concern is appropriate and surely widely experienced.

Third, keep your nerves at bay with the comforting thought that you have a timetable and are keeping up with it – it is rare that such a methodical approach will not be rewarded with success.

Inevitably you will get bored or stale. This is normal and decisive action is required because you may waste days in inefficient work. The remedy is a break for the evening or indeed a day. You will, however, have to be sparing with such breaks; remember the adage, 'think of ease but work on!' Don't neglect your sleep; for most people there is a direct relationship between sleep and productivity. The well-rested mind is more receptive, alert and retentive. Avoid getting overtired and inefficient, especially towards the end of the revision period. If you can add in regular exercise so much the better.

Linking with a supportive friend also sitting the examination can be helpful – in isolation perspective can be lost. Share any concerns you have – a problem shared is often a problem halved.

Revision course or not?

The majority of candidates will have some form of membership teaching course in their locality and some a revision course too. Revision courses are generally advantageous, though it is well worth you researching the options carefully before choosing a course. Talk to any colleagues who have recently taken their Part I and find out about the relative merits of the different courses. Remember that the better known residential courses may be booked up early, so it is sensible to give this matter your early attention. Much more will be gained from a course if you have virtually completed your revision and consequently many residential courses happen quite close to the examinations. It follows that it is ideal to build the revision course into your revision scheme when you are initially organizing yourself. Take your books with you and try to read up the topics on the day they are taught. Don't allow yourself to be unsettled by others on these courses – everyone will be knowledgeable in the area they are revising! A course offering MCQ and oral mocks is of especial value, though you can often organize these at your own hospital with a little perseverance. The best-known national courses are advertised in the *British Medical Journal* and the organizers are usually pleased to answer any queries you may have. Such courses include those held at the Institute of Psychiatry, London and at the University of Surrey, Guildford.

How to approach the last 2 weeks?

As mentioned earlier, it is ideal to have completed your revision about 2 weeks before the examinations. In the last 2 weeks review areas of difficulty, look through any notes you have highlighted for final revision and rehearse your clinical and MCQ examination technique. You should review your MCQ technique and sit more practice papers under examination conditions. Don't work late into the night in a frantic attempt to cram in more facts – the syllabus is virtually infinite, but your cognitive powers are not. Try to keep a sensible perspective on this. Good luck!

Summary

1. It is ideal to approach your revision with a foundation of steady learning behind you. Start your revision in good time and aim to

leave some time over before the examinations for more leisurely final revision.
2. Stick to a small number of core texts and journals but know them thoroughly.
3. Integrate your revision for the Part I examination within a well-organized timetable. Set yourself deadlines and keep to them.
4. Do large numbers of MCQs, especially as complete papers under examination conditions. Make brief notes of new pieces of information.
5. Give time and thought to your psychological preparation. Above all, avoid getting overtired and inefficient.
6. It is advantageous, but not essential, to attend a revision course. Leave time for this in your timetable, completing most of your revision before you arrive on the course.
7. Use your last 2 weeks to consolidate your learning. Avoid working up to the last minute and keep yourself fresh.

Before the examination – how best to make your final preparations?

Give some forethought to the examination day. It is reasonable to stop your revision the afternoon before and to relax in the evening. Have an early night.

Should you take any medication?

The use at examinations of beta-blockers such as propranolol and anxiolytics such as diazepam is ideally avoided. However, if you feel you are excessively anxious about the examinations and such anxiety has impaired your performance in the past, it seems very reasonable to discuss this with your general practitioner. Do so in good time. If you are to have medication, determine the influence of it on your performance well before the examinations.

If you tend to sleep badly the night before an examination – perhaps tossing and turning all night, unable to 'switch off' – it is advisable to find a solution before the date. Such insomnia masquerades as anxiety and worry, yet is often more a product of excessive caffeine consumption. If this is the cause, reduce gradually and in good time. If caffeine is not the explanation, you may need to consider a hypnotic, selecting one from the malted drink–alcohol–antihistamine–benzodiazepine range. Be aware of the hangover effects of any hypnotic drugs and make sure you don't oversleep.

What should be taken to the examinations and what to leave behind?

It is advisable to take a good rubber and two 2B pencils to the examination. Ensure you have a reliable watch with which to gauge your progress. Bring your letter from the Royal College containing your examination instructions and candidate number.

Don't take notes and papers with you – this is being excessive and is unlikely to be of any significant value. Give that memory of yours a little credence. If there are really one or two *small* points you find hard to remember, jot them down, read them before you go to bed, glance at them on waking and then drop them in a bin before you get to the examination venue.

How to organize your travel arrangements?

Ensure you don't oversleep; consider investing in a telephone alarm-call as a back-up to your own alarm. Arrive at the examination hall in good time – it is unsettling to arrive with only minutes to spare, and if you are late, you may not be admitted.

What to do when you get to the examination centre?

If you find the *bonhomie* outside examination halls unsettling, do not be afraid to detach yourself from this; find a quiet corner where you can contemplate your method or just distract yourself, perhaps with a newspaper. It can be a useful distraction to go to the cloakroom to freshen yourself up. A cup of tea or coffee can have the same effect, though beware the diuretic effect!

How to get yourself into a good frame of mind for the examination?

As a good psychiatrist you should not neglect your mental preparation. Think positively. Think of past triumphs, not misfortunes. Be determined and have a fighting spirit; stick up for yourself! Remind yourself that it is normal to feel some apprehension. Don't allow your resolve to be deflected by the outward manner of others. Don't panic when you hear someone pontificating about an obscurity that they have recently looked up. If you are to concentrate on anything, just remind yourself of a few of the tips listed below. Better, however, is to read your newspaper, look at the plants, contemplate the pictures or plan a treat for yourself on the way home.

Summary

1 Don't work until the last minute.
2. Prepare your travel arrangements carefully. Take a few essential items.
3. Deal with anxiety and sleeplessness in good time.
4. Plan your activity while you wait to enter the examination hall.
5. Actively prepare yourself mentally. Be determined and think positively.

In the examination – how best to approach doing the MCQ paper?

Well, the moment has arrived. The paper is in front of you! You could just turn up to do it, but why not enhance your potential with a little foresight?

Some general points

Do take the trouble to read over the instructions, however familiar they may appear. Ensure you understand how many questions there are to do in what period (in the MRCPsych Part I this should be 50 questions in 90 minutes). Set your watch to monitor your progress.

As you go through the paper ensure you have placed your answers on the response sheet in the correct place; if you miss a question out there is a risk of muddling up the subsequent numbering. Check that all your responses are clearly marked in the spaces provided (lozenges).

Which method to employ in answering the questions?

As there is no fixed pass mark your objective is to score as many marks as possible. Thus, don't stop when you believe you have correctly answered enough to score at a hypothetical pass mark. Work on until you find that to attempt any more would demand imprudent guessing. The author finds the best technique is to work through the paper, first answering those items that one is sure of. This has the advantage of getting a reasonable number of marks 'in the bag' and allows time to reflect more deeply on those items for which the correct answers are not so immediately obvious. Be careful, however; if your initial run through the paper is too hurried you will make costly slips, so be sure to read each question carefully on the first run. Some candidates find this approach less satisfactory, finding it better to do each question more thoroughly, thereby finishing without time for a major run back through the paper. Each approach should have been tried out with practice MCQ papers under examination conditions before the examination to ensure that the most suitable method is used on the day.

How to answer difficult questions – should I guess?

A lot is written about this issue. The dilemma is that an incorrect response to an item will lose a mark, whereas leaving the item out will result in no such penalty. The answer is really quite simple. *You should guess if you feel relatively certain you are correct. Though some of these guesses may be wrong, sufficient will be right to raise your score overall. If you really have no idea, then there is no advantage to be gained from guessing as you are just as likely to be wrong as right and may very well lose marks overall.* Thus, on each item where you find yourself uncertain, ask yourself, 'Is this a blind guess or is it an informed, reasoned one?' You have to be scrupulously honest with yourself when doing this.

Your MCQ practice should include time spent doing an examination three times as follows: first, answering all the questions; second, only answering those you are sure of; third, answering all those you are sure of and all those that you can take an informed guess at, possibly aided by clues gleaned from the MCQ technique discussed in the earlier sections. From this you can see how well you are guessing and your approach should be adjusted accordingly.

While the reckless guesser will clearly be penalized, it has been shown that the overcautious candidate who, having failed previously to assess the advantage of informed guessing, avoids even reasoned guessing (Fleming, 1988).

Summary

1. Read the examination instructions carefully and set your watch to monitor your progress.
2. Always check that you have placed your answers on the response sheet correctly and ensure that the lozenges are clearly marked.
3. Read the items carefully. Use the technique for answering the questions which previous rehearsal has shown suits you best.
4. Ensure you can differentiate in your mind an uninformed guess from a reasoned, informed one.
5. Avoid rash, uninformed guessing; this is likely to result in marks being deducted from your complete total. Be sure to use reasoned guesses and gauge the accuracy of your guessing when doing practice questions.

Résumé – 20 steps to ensure you pass the examination

A résumé of the previous advice on how to pass the examination is provided in the following 20 steps, which, for clarity, are divided into a first section on preparation and a second on sitting the examination.

Preparation for the examination

1. Write to the Royal College early in your training, well before the examination. Familiarize yourself with the examination regulations and guidelines.
2. Check the application dates well in advance. Identify your sponsors and ensure your application is lodged with the College in good time.
3. Work steadily through your training, looking up areas you are unsure of as they arise.
4. Organize your revision time very thoroughly. Set deadlines and keep to them.
5. Consider carefully the potential advantages of a revision course and, if you decide to attend one, integrate it into your programme, completing most of your revision before you arrive.
6. When you commence your revision in earnest keep to a core group of texts.
7. Complement your reading and learning with practice in all sections of the examination. Do a large number of MCQs. Ensure a proportion of your practice is with complete papers under strict examination conditions. Develop a system for pacing yourself for the 50 questions in 90 minutes.
8. Ensure you know the principles used to set MCQs and give careful consideration to your answering technique (see below). In particular, assess your ability to guess by doing a practice paper in three ways: first, answering all the questions; second, answering only those you are sure about; and third, taking informed guesses where you can. Use this to guide your subsequent guessing.
9. Give careful thought to your well-being as you revise. Above all, avoid getting overtired and inefficient. If you anticipate needing medication for insomnia or anxiety, don't take the first dose in the week of your examination – understand its impact before then.
10. Plan your journey to the examination carefully and ensure you don't oversleep. Arrive in good time. Bring a few essential items. Avoid last-minute cramming. In particular, prepare yourself mentally – be determined and think positively.

Sitting the examination

1. Read the examination instructions carefully and set your watch to monitor your progress. Allocate your time carefully.
2. Read each question item carefully. Regard each item as independent. Work fast but cautiously: (a) concentrate on the meaning; (b) watch for negatives; (c) watch for words that can be misread (e.g. cataplexy for catalepsy); (d) note terminology such as characteristic, recognized, typical, etc.; (e) watch for grammatical clues, especially absolutes such as never and always, which tend to be False, and watch out for the term 'may'.
3. Try to obtain the highest score you can without rash guessing. Use a predetermined approach to answering the questions – most candidates first answer those questions they are certain of, returning to ponder those left out.
4. Think round questions that are not immediately answerable, e.g. consider the implication if the answer were True or False, think about related conditions, and so on. Do use informed, reasoned guessing or you may underscore.
5. Try not leave out all the items on a question; there should be one that is answerable. Don't give in too easily. Don't get alarmed if you can't recall a well-known fact; return to the item later.
6. Take care not to muddle the numbering on the response sheet, especially if you first mark the question sheet and later transcribe the answers to the response sheet (transcribing your answers like this is not recommended).
7. Don't overread the questions, thereby creating ambiguities that don't exist. Take them at face value and trust the examiner. If they are truly ambiguous, leave them out; remember their interpretation will be difficult for other candidates too.
8. Watch our for any absurd or far-fetched details that suggest the item is a distractor. Look for items within the same question that may be interrelated and provide a lead.
9. Check that you have marked the lozenges on the response sheet clearly. Ensure that you have not filled in two lozenges for a single question item.
10. Never leave early – use any spare time at the end to check you have not muddled your numbering, misread any of the question wording and so on. Be wary of altering lots of your original responses; with informed guesses, your first inclinations tend to be more often correct.

References

American Psychiatric Association (1994) *Diagnostic and Statistical Manual of Mental Disorders*, 4th edn. (DSM–IV). Washington DC: APA.

Anderson, J. (1976) *The Multiple Choice Question in Medicine*. Tunbridge Wells: Pitman Medical.

Anderson, J. (1979) For multiple choice questions. *Medical Teacher* **1**, 37.

Anderson, J. (1981) The MCQ controversy – a review. *Medical Teacher* **3**, 150–156.

Bisson, J.I. (1991) The psychiatric MCQ: are 'possibles' always true? *Psychiatric Bulletin* **15**, 90–91.

Fish, F. (1985) *Clinical Psychopathology: Signs and Symptoms in Psychiatry*, 2nd edn. (Hamilton, M., ed). Bristol: Wright.

Fleming, P.R. (1988) The profitability of 'guessing' in multiple choice question papers. *Medical Education* **22**, 509–513.

Gelder, M., Gath, D. & Mayou, R. (1989) *Oxford Textbook of Psychiatry*, 2nd edn. Oxford: Oxford University Press.

Institute of Psychiatry, Department of Psychiatry (1987) *Notes on Eliciting and Recording Clinical Information in Psychiatric Patients*, 2nd edn. Oxford: Oxford University Press.

Kendell, R. E. & Zealley, A. K. (1993) *Companion to Psychiatric Studies*, 5th edn. Edinburgh: Churchill Livingstone.

Kräupl-Taylor, F. (1979) *Psychopathology: Its causes and symptoms*, revised edn. Sunbury-on-Thames: Quartermaine House.

Lowe, D. (1991) How to do it: set a multiple choice question (MCQ) examination. *British Medical Journal* **302**, 780–782.

Morgan, H.G. & Hill, P.D. (1991) MCQs in the MRCPsych examinations. *Psychiatric Bulletin* **15**, 108.

Pickering, G. (1979) Against multiple choice questions. *Medical Teacher* **1**, 84.

Royal College of Psychiatrists (1993) *General Information and Regulations for the MRCPsych Examinations*. London: Royal College of Psychiatrists.

Silverstone, T. & Turner, P. (1988) *Drug Treatments in Psychiatry*, 4th edn. London: Routledge.

Sims, A. (1988) *Symptoms in the Mind*. London: Baillière Tindall.

Slade, P.D. & Dewey, M.E. (1983) Role of grammatical clues in multiple choice questions: an empirical study. *Medical Teacher* **5**, 146–148.

Smyth, M.G. (1991) MCQs: a suggested study technique. *Psychiatric Bulletin* **15**, 88–90.

Strauss, G.D., Yager, J. & Strauss, G.E. (1982) Assessing assessment: the content and quality of the psychiatry in-training examination. *American Journal of Psychiatry* **139**, 85–88.

World Health Organization (1992) *The ICD-10 Classification of Mental and Behavioural Disorders*. Geneva: World Health Organization.

Section II:

Sample examination response sheets

PSYCHIATRY

Examination Answer Sheet

Surname

Initials

Examination Paper

Identification Code

<0>	<0>	<0>	<0>	<0>	<0>
<1>	<1>	<1>	<1>	<1>	<1>
<2>	<2>	<2>	<2>	<2>	<2>
<3>	<3>	<3>	<3>	<3>	<3>
<4>	<4>	<4>	<4>	<4>	<4>
<5>	<5>	<5>	<5>	<5>	<5>
<6>	<6>	<6>	<6>	<6>	<6>
<7>	<7>	<7>	<7>	<7>	<7>
<8>	<8>	<8>	<8>	<8>	<8>
<9>	<9>	<9>	<9>	<9>	<9>

Please use 2B PENCIL only. Rub out all errors thoroughly.
Mark lozenges like ⬬ NOT like this ✓ ✗ ⊖

T ⬭ = True F ⬭ = False DK ⬭ = Don't Know

	A	B	C	D	E
1	T ⬭ F ⬭ DK ⬭	T ⬭ F ⬭ DK ⬭	T ⬭ F ⬭ DK ⬭	T ⬭ F ⬭ DK ⬭	T ⬭ F ⬭ DK ⬭
2	T ⬭ F ⬭ DK ⬭	T ⬭ F ⬭ DK ⬭	T ⬭ F ⬭ DK ⬭	T ⬭ F ⬭ DK ⬭	T ⬭ F ⬭ DK ⬭
3	T ⬭ F ⬭ DK ⬭	T ⬭ F ⬭ DK ⬭	T ⬭ F ⬭ DK ⬭	T ⬭ F ⬭ DK ⬭	T ⬭ F ⬭ DK ⬭
4	T ⬭ F ⬭ DK ⬭	T ⬭ F ⬭ DK ⬭	T ⬭ F ⬭ DK ⬭	T ⬭ F ⬭ DK ⬭	T ⬭ F ⬭ DK ⬭
5	T ⬭ F ⬭ DK ⬭	T ⬭ F ⬭ DK ⬭	T ⬭ F ⬭ DK ⬭	T ⬭ F ⬭ DK ⬭	T ⬭ F ⬭ DK ⬭
6	T ⬭ F ⬭ DK ⬭	T ⬭ F ⬭ DK ⬭	T ⬭ F ⬭ DK ⬭	T ⬭ F ⬭ DK ⬭	T ⬭ F ⬭ DK ⬭
7	T ⬭ F ⬭ DK ⬭	T ⬭ F ⬭ DK ⬭	T ⬭ F ⬭ DK ⬭	T ⬭ F ⬭ DK ⬭	T ⬭ F ⬭ DK ⬭
8	T ⬭ F ⬭ DK ⬭	T ⬭ F ⬭ DK ⬭	T ⬭ F ⬭ DK ⬭	T ⬭ F ⬭ DK ⬭	T ⬭ F ⬭ DK ⬭
9	T ⬭ F ⬭ DK ⬭	T ⬭ F ⬭ DK ⬭	T ⬭ F ⬭ DK ⬭	T ⬭ F ⬭ DK ⬭	T ⬭ F ⬭ DK ⬭
10	T ⬭ F ⬭ DK ⬭	T ⬭ F ⬭ DK ⬭	T ⬭ F ⬭ DK ⬭	T ⬭ F ⬭ DK ⬭	T ⬭ F ⬭ DK ⬭

	A	B	C	D	E
11	T ⬭ F ⬭ DK ⬭	T ⬭ F ⬭ DK ⬭	T ⬭ F ⬭ DK ⬭	T ⬭ F ⬭ DK ⬭	T ⬭ F ⬭ DK ⬭
12	T ⬭ F ⬭ DK ⬭	T ⬭ F ⬭ DK ⬭	T ⬭ F ⬭ DK ⬭	T ⬭ F ⬭ DK ⬭	T ⬭ F ⬭ DK ⬭
13	T ⬭ F ⬭ DK ⬭	T ⬭ F ⬭ DK ⬭	T ⬭ F ⬭ DK ⬭	T ⬭ F ⬭ DK ⬭	T ⬭ F ⬭ DK ⬭
14	T ⬭ F ⬭ DK ⬭	T ⬭ F ⬭ DK ⬭	T ⬭ F ⬭ DK ⬭	T ⬭ F ⬭ DK ⬭	T ⬭ F ⬭ DK ⬭
15	T ⬭ F ⬭ DK ⬭	T ⬭ F ⬭ DK ⬭	T ⬭ F ⬭ DK ⬭	T ⬭ F ⬭ DK ⬭	T ⬭ F ⬭ DK ⬭
16	T ⬭ F ⬭ DK ⬭	T ⬭ F ⬭ DK ⬭	T ⬭ F ⬭ DK ⬭	T ⬭ F ⬭ DK ⬭	T ⬭ F ⬭ DK ⬭
17	T ⬭ F ⬭ DK ⬭	T ⬭ F ⬭ DK ⬭	T ⬭ F ⬭ DK ⬭	T ⬭ F ⬭ DK ⬭	T ⬭ F ⬭ DK ⬭
18	T ⬭ F ⬭ DK ⬭	T ⬭ F ⬭ DK ⬭	T ⬭ F ⬭ DK ⬭	T ⬭ F ⬭ DK ⬭	T ⬭ F ⬭ DK ⬭
19	T ⬭ F ⬭ DK ⬭	T ⬭ F ⬭ DK ⬭	T ⬭ F ⬭ DK ⬭	T ⬭ F ⬭ DK ⬭	T ⬭ F ⬭ DK ⬭
20	T ⬭ F ⬭ DK ⬭	T ⬭ F ⬭ DK ⬭	T ⬭ F ⬭ DK ⬭	T ⬭ F ⬭ DK ⬭	T ⬭ F ⬭ DK ⬭

PLEASE TURN OVER

Side 2

	A	B	C	D	E
21	T F DK	T F DK	T F DK	T F DK	T F DK
22	T F DK	T F DK	T F DK	T F DK	T F DK
23	T F DK	T F DK	T F DK	T F DK	T F DK
24	T F DK	T F DK	T F DK	T F DK	T F DK
25	T F DK	T F DK	T F DK	T F DK	T F DK
26	T F DK	T F DK	T F DK	T F DK	T F DK
27	T F DK	T F DK	T F DK	T F DK	T F DK
28	T F DK	T F DK	T F DK	T F DK	T F DK
29	T F DK	T F DK	T F DK	T F DK	T F DK
30	T F DK	T F DK	T F DK	T F DK	T F DK
31	T F DK	T F DK	T F DK	T F DK	T F DK
32	T F DK	T F DK	T F DK	T F DK	T F DK
33	T F DK	T F DK	T F DK	T F DK	T F DK
34	T F DK	T F DK	T F DK	T F DK	T F DK
35	T F DK	T F DK	T F DK	T F DK	T F DK

	A	B	C	D	E
36	T F DK	T F DK	T F DK	T F DK	T F DK
37	T F DK	T F DK	T F DK	T F DK	T F DK
38	T F DK	T F DK	T F DK	T F DK	T F DK
39	T F DK	T F DK	T F DK	T F DK	T F DK
40	T F DK	T F DK	T F DK	T F DK	T F DK
41	T F DK	T F DK	T F DK	T F DK	T F DK
42	T F DK	T F DK	T F DK	T F DK	T F DK
43	T F DK	T F DK	T F DK	T F DK	T F DK
44	T F DK	T F DK	T F DK	T F DK	T F DK
45	T F DK	T F DK	T F DK	T F DK	T F DK
46	T F DK	T F DK	T F DK	T F DK	T F DK
47	T F DK	T F DK	T F DK	T F DK	T F DK
48	T F DK	T F DK	T F DK	T F DK	T F DK
49	T F DK	T F DK	T F DK	T F DK	T F DK
50	T F DK	T F DK	T F DK	T F DK	T F DK

DRS Data & Research Services plc/H74240395/SRVK

Paper 1

1.1 Recognized causes of olfactory hallucinations include:

A. Depression.
B. Schizophrenia.
C. Obsessive-compulsive disorder.
D. Temporal lobe epilepsy.
E. Anorexia nervosa.

1.2 Flight of ideas is:

A. A form of thought disorder.
B. Characteristic of mania.
C. Loosening of associations.
D. Characterized by neologisms.
E. Characterized by verbigeration.

1.3 Delusional perception:

A. Is a disturbance of perception.
B. Is a disturbance of thought.
C. Is a form of delusion.
D. Is a form of idea of reference.
E. Is readily understood.

1.1

A. T – In depression olfactory hallucinations are typically of foul odour.
B. T – In schizophrenia they are often subordinate to hallucinations in other modalities. They may be the dominant complaint in late-onset paranoid schizophrenia.
C. F – Not described.
D. T – Olfactory hallucinations commonly form the aura in temporal lobe epilepsy.
E. F – Not described.

Further reading: Pryse-Phillips (1971); Meats (1988); Sims (1988; pp. 73–74)

1.2

A. T – Acceleration of the flow of thinking.
B. T.
C. F – The logical sequence of ideas is preserved and there is no loosening of associations, but the goal of thinking is not maintained for long.
D. F – Neologisms are characteristic of schizophrenia. Clang associations, punning, rhyming and responding to distracting cues in the immediate environment are characteristic of flight of ideas.
E. F – Verbigeration refers to a kind of stereotypy in which sounds, words, or pharases are repeated in a senseless way.

Further reading: Sims (1988; p. 108); Gelder *et al.* (1989; pp. 11–12)

1.3

A. F – Delusional perception is a disturbance of thought.
B. T – It occurs when some abnormal significance, usually with self-reference, is attached to a genuine perception without any justification.
C. T – First the object is perceived and then invested with delusional significance.
D. F – Ideas of reference have sufficient ground to explain them.
E. F – See B.

Further reading: Schneider (1959; pp. 104–107); Sims (1988; pp. 87–90)

1.4 Ecstasy:

A. Is a normal phenomenon.
B. May be seen in epilepsy.
C. Is a passivity experience.
D. May occur in hysterical dissociation.
E. May occur in alexithymia.

1.5 Illusions:

A. Are false perceptions.
B. Can occur during inattention.
C. Pareidolic illusions are banished by attention.
D. Are a feature of the Capgras syndrome.
E. Are a feature of temporal lobe epilepsy.

1.6 The following are true of confabulation:

A. Suggestibility is a prominent feature.
B. It is an impaired ability to learn or form new memories.
C. It is always a feature of Korsakoff's syndrome
D. Two forms have been described.
E. The patient gives an incoherent and false account of some recent event or experience.

1.4

A. T – But can occur in people with mental illness.
B. T – And in other organic states.
C. F – The change in ego boundaries in ecstasy does not have the characteristic of interference with self which accompanies passivity experiences.
D. T.
E. F – Individuals with alexithymia have difficulties in recognizing and describing their own feelings. They also have a diminished capacity for fantasy.

Further reading: Sims (1988; pp. 227–228)

1.5

A. T – Illusions, hallucinations and pseudohallucinations are false perceptions.
B. T – Completion and affect illusions occur during inattention. Pareidolic illusions can increase in intensity during attention.
C. F.
D. F – Although termed the illusion of doubles, the Capgras syndrome is not an illusion but a delusional misinterpretation.
E. T.

Further reading: Sims (1988; pp. 65–67)

1.6

A. T – This is a feature of all types of confabulation (Korsakoff syndrome, dementia and other organic states).
B. F – This is anterograde amnesia. Confabulation is a 'falsification of memory occurring in clear consciousness in association with an organically derived amnesia' (Berlyne, 1972).
C. F – It is often included in the definition of Korsakoff syndrome but only occurs in a proportion of these patients.
D. T – Two varieties, momentary and fantastic, have been described in Korsakoff syndrome. Fantastic confabulation occurs mainly in the initial phase and momentary confabulation occurs later.
E. F – The account is typically coherent.

Further reading: Berlyne (1972); Lishman (1987; pp. 29–30); Sims (1988; pp. 44–45); Adams and Victor (1989; pp. 341–342, 824)

1.7 Characteristic features of dissociative (hysterical, psychogenic) fugue states include:

A. Clouding of consciousness.
B. Memory loss.
C. Disturbed behaviour.
D. Duration of hours to weeks.
E. Sudden onset.

1.8 Pseudohallucinations:

A. Are located in outer objective space.
B. Are experienced as real or concrete.
C. Are created voluntarily.
D. Are pathognomonic of organic states.
E. Were first described by Jaspers.

1.9 The following statements about the superego are true:

A. Many of its functions are unconscious.
B. It incorporates the notion of an ego-ideal.
C. It is concerned with rational thinking.
D. Not all its operations are conscious.
E. It corresponds roughly to consciousness.

1.7

A. F – Dissociative fugue is characterized by dissociative amnesia, apparently purposeful travel beyond the usual everyday range, maintenance of self-care and simple interaction with strangers (*ICD-10*).
B. T – Dissociative amnesia.
C. F – Behaviour is usually appropriate and the individual appears to be in contact with his or her environment.
D. T – Duration is short.
E. T – Onset is typically sudden, in response to emotional stress.

Further reading: Gelder *et al.* (1989; p. 206); World Health Organization (1992)

1.8

A. F – Located in inner subjective space.
B. F – The experience is figurative, not concrete or real.
C. F – They are not created voluntarily.
D. F – They are not pathognomonic of any particular mental illness.
E. F – Coined by Kandinsky (1885), but discussed by Jaspers in his book *Allgemeine Psychopathologie* (1948, original 1913).

Further reading: Kräupl-Taylor (1981); Sims (1988; pp. 74–76)

1.9

A. T.
B. T – Two aspects of the superego can be distinguished – first, the punitive and primitive aspects and second, the more positive aspects of the ego-ideal.
C. F – The ego is concerned with rational thinking, external perception and voluntary motor function.
D. T.
E. F – The superego corresponds roughly to the conscience.

Further reading: Brown and Pedder (1991; pp. 46–48)

1.10 In psychoanalytic theory, the unconscious:

A. Disregards reality.
B. Is the origin of basic instinctual drives.
C. Is described in the structural model of the mind.
D. Includes memories of which we are not immediately aware, but which can be fairly easily brought to full consciousness.
E. Includes primitive impulses and fantasies.

1.11 The following statements are correct:

A. Bowlby considers the period from 9 months to 3 years the time of maximal attachment behaviour.
B. Piaget's developmental theory focuses on emotional development.
C. In Erikson's stages of psychosocial development, basic trust in others is laid down between the ages of 2 and 3.
D. Freud's Oedipal phase corresponds with Erikson's third stage of initiative versus guilt.
E. Borderline personality disorder is thought to result from disturbances in the earliest phase of development (0–1 year).

1.10

A. T – It disregards the reality of the conscious world.
B. T – These impulses or drives threaten the integrity and function of the other areas of the mind and must be kept in check. Freud initially regarded these drives as entirely sexual, but later placed more emphasis on aggressive impulses.
C. F – In psychoanalytic theory the unconscious is described in the topographical model of the mind, the other components being the preconscious and the conscious. The structural theory incorporates the superego, ego and id.
D. F – This describes the preconscious of the topographical model. The unconscious includes repressed memories and sensations which are not so readily available.
E. T.

Further reading: Gelder *et al.* (1989; pp. 119–123); Brown and Pedder (1991; pp. 14–20, 46–47)

1.11

A. T.
B. F – It focuses on cognitive and intellectual development: sensorimotor stage (0–2 years), preoperational thought (2–7 years), concrete thinking (7–11 years), abstract thinking (11+).
C. F – This is thought to occur in the first year of life.
D. T.
E. T.

Further reading: Brown and Pedder (1991; pp. 37–46)

1.12 The following terms are associated with Bion:

A. Common group tension.
B. Dependence.
C. Analysis through the group.
D. Pairing.
E. Cohesiveness.

1.13 The following are correctly paired:

A. Carl Rogers: Transactional Analysis.
B. Arthur Janov: 'Muscular Armour'.
C. Moreno: Psychodrama.
D. Main: Therapeutic Community.
E. Fritz Perls: Psychosynthesis.

1.12

A. F – Common group tension is an expression which was coined by Ezriel to describe the group conflict resulting from a shared, wished for, but avoided relationship with the therapist.
B. T – Dependence, fight–flight and pairing are Bion's three basic assumptions, or primitive states of mind which are generated automatically when people combine in a group.
C. F – Analysis through the group is associated with Foulkes. Bion and Ezriel were interested in analysis of the group.
D. T.
E. F – Cohesiveness is one of the several therapeutic factors specific to groups described by Yalom.

Further reading: Yalom (1985); Brown and Pedder (1991; pp. 121–123, 133)

1.13

A. F – Carl Rogers developed client-centred therapy and the Encounter Movement. Transactional Analysis was founded by Eric Berne.
B. F – Arthur Janov developed Primal Therapy, an emotional release therapy. Wilhelm Reich developed the idea of 'Muscular Armour' (body armour) and organ energy accumulator. This has developed into bioenergetics.
C. T – Moreno developed the approach of Psychodrama.
D. T – Tom Main first made use of the term in 1946.
E. F – Fritz Perls described Gestalt therapy, which draws on Gestalt psychology, psychodrama, existentialism and psychoanalysis.

Further reading: Clare (1993; pp. 882–885)

1.14 The following statements about Melanie Klein's theory are correct:

A. Forerunners of the superego are demonstrable during the first 2 years of life.
B. The important drives are sexual ones.
C. Children can only be analysed from 3 years.
D. The paranoid-schizoid position occupies the first 6 months.
E. She did not accept orthodox Freudian theory.

1.15 Persisting cognitive impairment after head injury:

A. Typically occurs when there is post-traumatic amnesia of between 12 and 24 hours.
B. Is more likely with increasing age.
C. Usually improves substantially during the first 6 months after injury.
D. Is more likely following damage to the non-dominant hemisphere.
E. Is in proportion to the amount of damage to the brain.

1.14

A. T – Kleinian theory traces the origins of the superego back to the earliest months of life. Orthodox Freudian theory accepts that the superego arises during the fourth year.
B. F – This is the more orthodox Freudian theory. Klein believed that the important drives are aggressive ones.
C. F – Klein treated children as young as 2 years using a method centred around the fantasy life of the child as revealed in play. The cooperation of the parents was not sought.
D. T – The baby's notions of aggression are conditioned by the fact that it is at the oral stage of development.
E. F – Klein accepted orthodox Freudian theory but claimed to have opened up unexplored regions in the pre-Oedipal stages.

Further reading: Brown (1961; pp. 73–77)

1.15

A. F – Usually occurs when the duration of post-traumatic amnesia is more than 24 hours for a closed head injury. The length of post-traumatic amnesia is a less reliable guide in penetrating injuries. In a closed head injury, if the post-traumatic amnesia is under 24 hours, a complete intellectual recovery should be expected in a fair proportion of cases.
B. T.
C. T – Though during subsequent years further improvement can occur.
D. F – Intellectual impairment is more likely following damage to the dominant lobe.
E. T.

Further reading: Lishman (1987; pp. 156–157)

1.16 The differential diagnosis of Huntington's chorea includes:
A. Inherited cerebellar ataxia.
B. Creutzfeldt–Jakob disease.
C. Wilson's disease.
D. Choreoacanthocytosis.
E. Parkinson's disease.

1.17 Characteristic features of Wernicke's encephalopathy include:
A. Ataxia.
B. Confusion.
C. Amblyopia.
D. Ophthalmoplegia.
E. Intention tremor.

1.18 The following features are characteristic of frontal lobe syndrome:
A. *Witzelsucht.*
B. Impaired judgement.
C. Lack of initiative and spontaneity.
D. Prosopagnosia.
E. Constructional apraxia.

1.16

A. T – May present as an autosomal dominant disease and be difficult to differentiate from Huntington's in the early stages.
B. T – But the rapid downhill course of Creutzfeldt–Jakob disease differentiates it from Huntington's chorea.
C. T – Occurs at a young age (autosomal recessive).
D. T – Autosomal recessive.
E. T – But non-progressive and no family history.

Further reading: Martin (1984); Lishman (1987; pp. 393–400)

1.17

A. T – The classical triad includes confusion, ataxia and ophthalmoplegia. Ataxia can be very severe in the acute stages, but lesser degrees can also occur.
B. T.
C. F – In rare cases retrobulbar neuritis may develop in alcoholics and is associated with peripheral neuropathy. Deficiencies of thiamine and B_{12} appear to be responsible.
D. T – Commonly, horizontal and vertical nystagmus, and bilateral weakness or paralysis of the lateral rectus muscles and weakness of conjugate gaze.
E. F – May occur but is relatively rare. If present it is more likely to be brought out by heel-to-knee than by finger-to-nose testing.

Further reading: Lishman (1987; pp. 491–500); Adams and Victor (1989; pp. 200, 822)

1.18

A. T – A tendency to prankish joking and punning.
B. T.
C. T.
D. F – This is defective recognition for faces and is associated with bilateral lesions of the ventromedial occipitotemporal regions.
E. F – Inability to reproduce geometric figures – seen in lesions of the parietal lobe, and more common and severe with lesions of the right lobe.

Further reading: Lishman (1987; pp. 68–71); Adams and Victor (1989; pp. 352–359)

1.19 The following hallucinations suggest a diagnosis of schizophrenia:

A. Third person auditory hallucinations.
B. Second person auditory hallucinations.
C. Voices echoing the patient's thoughts.
D. Visual hallucinations.
E. Tactile hallucinations.

1.20 The Capgras syndrome:

A. Is sometimes called *l'illusion des sosies*.
B. Is an illusion.
C. Is commoner in men than in women.
D. Is usually associated with epilepsy.
E. May have an organic component.

1.21 The following neurological abnormalities have been detected in schizophrenic patients:

A. Ventricular enlargement.
B. Thickening of the corpus callosum (CC).
C. Abnormalities in proprioception.
D. Peripheral neuropathy.
E. Sensory inattention.

1.19

A. T.
B. F – Second person auditory hallucinations of themselves do not point to a particular diagnosis, but their content and the patient's reaction can have diagnostic implications.
C. T – First-rank symptoms which suggest schizophrenia.
D. F – Visual hallucinations are more characteristic of organic disorders. They are uncommon in schizophrenia.
E. F – Not generally of diagnostic significance, but hallucinations of bodily sensation are quite common.

Further reading: Sims (1988; pp. 67–74); Gelder *et al.* (1989; pp. 9–10)

1.20

A. T.
B. F – Not an abnormality of perception but a delusional misidentification of a person or persons close to the patient.
C. F – Commoner in women.
D. F – Usually associated with schizophrenia or affective disorder.
E. T.

Further reading: Sims (1988; pp. 96–98); Gelder *et al.* (1989; p. 339)

1.21

A. T – Ventricular enlargement was first reported in air-encephalographic (EEG) studies and later confirmed in computed tomographic (CT) and magnetic resonance imaging (MRI) studies. It has been described in patients soon after the onset of schizophrenia and its significance is not understood.
B. T – Both abnormally thick and abnormally thin CC have been described in schizophrenia.
C. T – The commonest neurological 'soft' (non-localizing) signs reported in schizophrenia include stereognosis, graphaesthesia, balance and proprioception abnormalities.
D. F – This occurs in Korsakoff's syndrome.
E. F – Due to lesions in the parietal lobe.

Further reading: Gelder *et al.* (1989; pp. 298, 356–357); Coger and Serafetinides (1990)

1.22 Typical clinical features of the neuroleptic malignant syndrome include:

A. Muscle rigidity.
B. Akinetic mutism.
C. Autonomic disturbance.
D. Visual agnosia.
E. Cataplexy.

1.23 The following symptoms are more likely to be present in a schizophrenic psychosis than in an affective psychosis:

A. Perplexity.
B. Grandiose delusions.
C. Thought insertion.
D. Nihilistic delusions.
E. Incongruous affect.

1.22

A. T – The main clinical features of the neuroleptic malignant syndrome are motor, mental and autonomic. Motor symptoms include muscle rigidity in the muscles of the throat and chest. Mental symptoms include mutism, stupor and impaired consciousness. Hyperpyrexia and sweating also occur with autonomic disturbance. Neuroleptic malignant syndrome is a rare disorder and thought to be due to an idiosyncratic reaction to neuroleptic drugs.

B. T.

C. T.

D. F – This is a perceptual inability to identify an object by sight, despite an intact visual system and absence of aphasia.

E. F – This consists of episodes of sudden weakness that can be precipitated by heightened emotional states such as laughter. It is a flaccid paresis and accompanies narcolepsy. Do not confuse with catalepsy.

Further reading: Gelder *et al.* (1989; pp. 649–650)

1.23

A. T – Perplexity is more likely to be seen in a schizophrenic psychosis.

B. F.

C. T – Thought insertion, thought withdrawal and thought broadcasting are all more likely to occur in a schizophrenic psychosis, although they have been described in conjunction with affective psychoses.

D. F.

E. T.

Further reading: Kendall (1993; pp. 401–402)

1.24 The differential diagnosis of neuroleptic malignant syndrome includes:

A. Lethal catatonia.
B. *Clostridium tetani* infection.
C. Malignant hyperpyrexia.
D. Encephalitis.
E. Phaeochromocytoma.

1.25 The following social circumstances put people at risk for a pathological grief reaction:

A. Supportive family.
B. Immigrant.
C. Employed.
D. Having dependent children.
E. Low socioeconomic status.

1.24

A. T – Characteristic features of lethal catatonia include hyperthermia, autonomic dysfunction and extrapyramidal effects, but there is also intense motor excitement, violent destructive behaviour, thought disorder and auditory and visual hallucinations.

B. T – Features of *Clostridium tetani* infection include hyperthermia, autonomic lability, sialorrhoea, rigidity, opisthotonos, trismus and diaphoresis. Between attacks there is a normal mental state and clear consciousness.

C. T – Malignant hyperpyrexia is an inherited muscle disorder in which general anaesthesia leads to widespread rhabdomyolysis, hyperpyrexia, muscle contraction, delirium, tachycardia and raised creatine kinase levels. The fever is less marked and the muscle necrosis less clear than in neuroleptic malignant syndrome.

D. T – Encephalitis must be ruled out, as must hallucinogen ingestion and delirium tremens.

E. F – In phaeochromocytoma, attacks are caused by tumours secreting adrenaline and noradrenaline, and are characterized by palpitations, blushing, sweating, tremulousness and violent headaches; also hypertension and tachycardia.

Further reading: Mann *et al.* (1986); Addonizio *et al.* (1987); Gibb (1988); Gelder *et al.* (1989; pp. 649–650, 382); Keck *et al.* (1989)

1.25

A. F – An absent or unsupportive family is a risk factor.

B. T – They are detached from traditional religious and cultural support systems.

C. F – Unemployment or unhappiness at work are risk factors.

D. T.

E. T.

Further reading: Parkes CM (1985).

1.26 The following are common features of a normal grief reaction:

A. Motor restlessness.
B. Suicidal thoughts.
C. Poor concentration.
D. Guilt about past actions.
E. Brief hallucinations.

1.27 Examples of Beck's cognitive distortions include:

A. Arbitrary interference.
B. Overgeneralization.
C. Ambivalence.
D. Selective abreaction.
E. Depersonalization.

1.26

A. T – Sadness, weeping, poor sleep, loss of appetite, motor restlessness, poor concentration and memory are all characteristic features of a normal grief reaction.
B. F – These are uncommon, as are retardation and guilt about past actions in general.
C. T.
D. F.
E. T – One in 10 bereaved individuals report brief hallucinations and many have the experience that they are in the presence of the dead person.

Further reading: Parkes CM (1985); Gelder *et al.* (1989; pp. 226–227)

1.27

A. F – Arbitrary inference – drawing a conclusion when there is no evidence for it.
B. T – Drawing a general conclusion on the basis of a single incident.
C. F.
D. F – Selective abstraction – focusing on a detail and ignoring more important features of the situation.
E. F – Personalization – relating external events to oneself in an unwarranted way.

Note: The remaining cognitive distortions include minimization (underestimation of the individual's performance, achievement or ability) and magnification (inflation of the magnitude of the individual's problems).

Further reading: Beck (1967; pp. 228–240); Gelder *et al.* (1989; p. 737)

1.28 The following are true of puerperal psychosis:

A. It is more frequent in women with a family history of mental illness.
B. About half the cases are affective.
C. Onset is acute.
D. There are no differences in symptoms between puerperal psychosis and other psychoses.
E. There is a clear association between the psychosis and obstetric factors.

1.29 Characteristic features of 'winter-onset' seasonal affective disorder (SAD) include:

A. Early morning wakening.
B. Nihilistic delusions.
C. Weight loss.
D. Agitation.
E. Occurs equally in men and women.

1.30 The following physical illnesses are particularly associated with depression:

A. Parkinson's disease.
B. Hyperthyroidism.
C. Cushing's syndrome.
D. Influenza.
E. Infectious mononucleosis.

1.28

A. T – Also more frequent in primiparous women, those with a history of a major psychiatric illness and unmarried mothers.
B. F – 80% of cases are affective. Schizophrenic and organic syndromes also occur.
C. T – And usually in the first 2 weeks after delivery.
D. F – While manic syndromes are similar, puerperal major depressives show more delusions, hallucinations, disorientation, agitation and emotional lability.
E. F.

Further reading: Protheroe (1969); Dean and Kendall (1981); Platz and Kendall (1988)

1.29

A. F – Hypersomnia and increased sleep time are characteristic.
B. F.
C. F – Appetite is increased, with carbohydrate craving and weight gain.
D. F – Fatigue is characteristic.
E. F – Occurs mainly in women between 20 and 40 years.

Further reading: Rosenthal *et al.* (1984); Gelder *et al.* (1989; p. 230); Easton (1990)

1.30

A. T – This association is well-established.
B. F – Symptoms of hyperthyroidism may resemble anxiety, though depression may occur in a minority of patients.
C. T – Depressive symptoms are the most common psychiatric symptoms in Cushing's syndrome.
D. T.
E. T.

Further reading: Gelder *et al.* (1989; pp. 243, 379–391, 403–404)

1.31 Characteristic features of schizotypal personality disorder (DSM-IV) include:

A. Delusions of reference.
B. Suspiciousness.
C. Impulsiveness.
D. Odd speech.
E. Perfectionism.

1.32 Obsessive-compulsive personality disorder is:

A. Included in *ICD-10*.
B. Associated with secondary depression.
C. Rare.
D. Associated with a relatively high incidence of psychosis.
E. A chronic disorder.

1.31

A. F – Ideas of reference.
B. T.
C. F – A feature of antisocial personality disorder and borderline personality disorder.
D. T.
E. F – A feature of obsessive-compulsive personality disorder.

Further reading: American Psychiatric Association (1994)

1.32

A. F – It is included in *DSM-IV.* The *ICD-10* equivalent is anankastic personality disorder.
B. T – The clinical association between obsessive-compulsive disorder and depression is well-recognized; comorbid secondary depression is not uncommon.
C. F – It is more common than once believed.
D. T – Reactive affective or paranoid psychoses have been reported in follow-up studies of patients with obsessive-compulsive disease. These are generally transient.
E. T.

Further reading: Insel and Akiskal (1986); McDougle and Goodman (1990, 1991); World Health Organization (1992)

1.33 Clinical features of acute stress reactions (*ICD-10*) typically include:

A. Stupor.
B. Agitation.
C. Fugue.
D. Delusions.
E. Catatonia.

1.34 Simple phobias:

A. Are commoner in men.
B. Mostly arise *de novo* in adulthood.
C. Are best treated by relaxation training.
D. Typically lead to symptoms of depersonalization.
E. Are associated with mitral valve prolapse.

1.33

A. T – Some individuals develop characteristic symptoms following a major stressful event. Typically they seem dazed and may show some degree of disorientation and restricted response to their surroundings. They may also lapse into a stupor.

B. T – Purposeless activity and agitation have also been described.

C. T – They may also wander away from the stressful situation in a fugue-like state; symptoms usually start within minutes or hours of the stress and resolve over the next 2–3 days; there is no evidence of psychiatric disorder in the individuals prior to the stressful event.

D. F.

E. F.

Further reading: Freeman (1993; p. 518); Gelder *et al.* (1989; p. 163); World Health Organization (1992)

1.34

A. F – Lifetime prevalence estimated at 4–15% for men and 9–26% for women.

B. F – Most simple phobias of adulthood are a continuation of childhood phobias. A minority begin in adult life, usually after stressful events.

C. F – Best treated by exposure techniques.

D. F – This is seen in association with agoraphobia.

E. F – An association has been reported between agoraphobia and prolapse of the mitral valve in women, but not confirmed in other studies.

Further reading: Gelder *et al.* (1989; pp. 183–191)

1.35 The following are true of compulsive rituals:
A. They are repetitive and seemingly purposeful behaviours.
B. They are never resisted.
C. They are usually associated with an obsession.
D. They are recognized as senseless.
E. Checking is commoner in women.

1.36 The following are characteristic features of the Ganser syndrome:
A. Approximate answers.
B. Dementia.
C. Somatic symptoms.
D. Delusions.
E. Clouding of consciousness.

1.35

A. T – They are performed in a stereotyped way.
B. F – Usually the individual has the urge to resist, but not always.
C. T – Compulsive rituals are repetitive acts based on obsessional thoughts and they are carried out in order to relieve the tension and anxiety caused by the obsessional thoughts.
D. T – This may be a more important criterion than resistance.
E. F – Washing is commoner in women. Checking is found equally in both sexes.

Further reading: Marks (1987; pp. 427–429); Freeman (1993; pp. 504–510); Gelder *et al.* (1989; pp. 22–24)

1.36

A. T – The patient's replies to questions are inaccurate and ridiculous. However, the answers usually approximate to the correct answers, indicating that the patient understood the purpose of the question.
B. F – The Ganser syndrome comes under the rubric of pseudodementia.
C. T – A large variety of symptoms has been described, including ataxia, difficulty in moving limbs, flaccidity or rigidity, headache, backache, analgesia or areas of anaesthesia. These are considered to be somatic conversion symptoms.
D. F – In Ganser's original series (1898), patients with prominent hallucinatory experiences were described. If hallucinations are present they are visual or auditory.
E. T – This is associated with perplexity. The complete syndrome is very rare. A distinction has been drawn between the Ganser symptom (approximate answers) and the Ganser syndrome.

Further reading: Enoch and Trethowan (1991; pp. 75–91); Lishman (1987; pp. 404–407)

1.37 Recognized features of agoraphobia include:

A. Panic attacks.
B. Occurs mainly in women.
C. Sufferers score highly in neuroticism questionnaires.
D. Depressive symptoms.
E. Depersonalization.

1.38 Gamma-aminobutyric acid (GABA):

A. Is an amino acid.
B. Is the principal inhibitory transmitter in the central nervous system (CNS).
C. Increased brain levels can cause convulsions.
D. Is present in the gastrointestinal tract.
E. Forms receptor complexes with tricyclic antidepressants.

1.37

A. T – Panic attacks are more common in agoraphobia than in other kinds of phobic disorder. The risk of panic attacks in first-degree relatives of agoraphobics and panic disorder patients has been shown to be roughly equal.
B. T – Agoraphobia occurs predominantly in women. Most cases begin in the early or middle 20s and there is a further period of high onset in the mid 30s.
C. T – Sufferers tend to be introverted.
D. T – These are common.
E. T – Depression, depersonalization and obsessional thoughts are more frequent in agoraphobia than in other phobic disorders.

Further reading: Freeman (1993); Gelder *et al.* (1989, pp. 186–190)

1.38

A. T – It is found widely in the CNS and acts as a postsynaptic inhibitory transmitter in the cerebral and cerebellar cortices. In the spinal cord it mediates postsynaptic inhibition of afferent pathways.
B. T.
C. F – A reduction in brain GABA levels may lead to convulsions. Inhibitors of GABA-transaminase, the enzyme that degrades GABA, have anticonvulsant activity.
D. F – It is restricted in its distribution to the CNS.
E. F – GABA forms complexes with benzodiazepines at various brain sites and these probably mediate the antianxiety, anticonvulsant, muscle relaxant and hypnotic effects of benzodiazepines.

Further reading: Reveley and Campbell (1984; pp. 74–75); Silverstone and Turner (1988; p. 16)

1.39 Dopamine:

A. Is a precursor in the synthetic pathway of noradrenaline.
B. Levels are depleted by reserpine.
C. Inhibits prolactin release.
D. Is a sympathomimetic amine.
E. Is a preferential substrate for monoamine oxidase MAO-A inhibition.

1.40 Akathisia:

A. Is characterized by choreiform movements.
B. Can present in a late-onset form.
C. Is effectively treated by anticholinergic drugs.
D. May improve with propranolol.
E. Is thought to be due to dopamine blockade in the nigrostriatal pathway.

1.39

A. T – Phenylalanine–tyrosine–dopa–dopamine–noradrenaline.
B. T – Reserpine is an alkaloid which depletes tissue stores of noradrenaline, dopamine, 5-hydroxytryptamine (5-HT) and histamine.
C. T – When dopamine is released from neurones of the hypothalamic–hypophyseal pathway, it inhibits prolactin release.
D. T – Dopamine, together with adrenaline, noradrenaline and isoprelanine, stimulates adrenergic receptors directly.
E. F – The MAO enzyme exists in two forms. MAO-A includes 5-HT and noradrenaline as its preferred substrates and MAO-B includes dopamine among its preferred substrates. Tyramine is a substrate for both.

Further reading: Silverstone and Turner (1988; pp. 13–15, 34–35)

1.40

A. F – This condition is characterized by motor restlessness, a subjective feeling of tension and an inability to tolerate inactivity, which gives rise to restless movement.
B. T – Acute akathisia occurs in some 20% of patients receiving antipsychotic drugs, usually within the first few days or weeks of treatment. A late-onset form also exists.
C. F – Anticholinergic drugs are ineffective in the majority of cases.
D. T.
E. F – Akathisia is thought to be due to blockade of dopamine receptors in the mesolimbic and mesocortical dopamine pathways.

Further reading: Silverstone and Turner (1988; pp. 126–127)

1.41 The following substances should be avoided during treatment with monoamine oxidase inhibitors (MAOIs):
A. Pethidine.
B. Lithium.
C. Imipramine.
D. Propranolol.
E. Ephedrine.

1.42 Early side-effects of lithium include:
A. Mild polyuria.
B. Nausea.
C. Constipation.
D. Hypothyroidism.
E. Benign and reversible depression of the T wave on the electrocardiogram (ECG).

1.43 The following drugs increase plasma levels of tricyclic antidepressants:
A. Antiepileptics.
B. Cimetidine.
C. Disulfiram.
D. Benzodiazepines.
E. Phenothiazines.

1.41

A. T – Pethidine is an opioid analgesic and, if given to patients on MAOIs, the combination can cause CNS excitation or depression (hypertension or hypotension).
B. F.
C. T – MAOIs, in combination with imipramine and other tricyclic antidepressants, can cause CNS excitation and hypertension.
D. F.
E. T – Ephedrine is a sympathomimetic and its effects are potentiated by MAOIs. Combination can cause hypertensive crisis.

Further reading: Baldessarini (1990; pp. 414–418); *British National Formulary* (1994; pp. 167–169)

1.42

A. T – Typically, mild polyuria appears early in treatment and then disappears. Late-developing polyuria is an indication to evaluate renal function, and is usually reversible.
B. T.
C. F – Usually diarrhoea.
D. F – Usually a late side-effect.
E. F – Again, usually a late side-effect.

Further reading: Baldessarini (1990; pp. 418–422)

1.43

A. F – Antiepileptics reduce plasma concentrations of tricyclics, thus causing a reduced antidepressant effect.
B. T – Plasma levels of amitriptyline, desipramine, doxepin, imipramine and nortriptyline are increased by cimetidine.
C. T – Disulfiram inhibits the metabolism of tricyclics.
D. F – No effect.
E. T – Chlorpromazine may block hydroxylation, therefore increasing plasma levels of tricyclics and potentiating their therapeutic action and side-effects.

Further reading: *British National Formulary* (1994; pp. 507–8)

1.44 Buspirone:
A. Has anxiolytic properties.
B. Is a benzodiazepine.
C. Is sedative.
D. Has anticonvulsant properties.
E. Has muscle relaxant properties.

1.45 The following statements are true:
A. Benzodiazepine agonists enhance the action of GABA.
B. Drugs causing a reduction in the action of GABA have an anxiolytic effect.
C. Benzodiazepine antagonists antagonize the actions of anxiolytic and anxiogenic compounds.
D. Benzodiazepine receptors are found only in the brain.
E. Clonazepam has a high affinity for the CNS benzodiazepine receptor.

1.46 Diencephalic structures include:
A. Thalamus.
B. Dentate nucleus.
C. Mamillary bodies.
D. Pineal body.
E. Amygdala.

1.47 The following cranial nerve nuclei are located in the medulla oblongata:
A. Abducens.
B. Hypoglossal.
C. Dorsal motor nucleus of vagus.
D. Facial.
E. Vestibular (inferior subnuclei).

1.44

A. T.
B. F.
C. F.
D. F – Lacks anticonvulsant and muscle relaxant properties.
E. F.

Further reading: Silverstone and Turner (1988; pp. 191–192)

1.45

A. T – And reduce anxiety.
B. F – These drugs, which are called benzodiazepine inverse agonists, increase anxiety.
C. T – eg. imidazodiazepine/flumazenil.
D. F – Peripheral benzodiazepine-binding sites have been identified and these are found outside and inside the CNS.
E. T.

Further reading: File (1988)

1.46

A. T – The diencephalon consists of four major components bilaterally – the thalamus (the largest component), subthalamus, epithalamus and hypothalamus.
B. F – The dentate nucleus is found in the cerebellum.
C. T – The mamillary bodies are located on the ventral surface of the hypothalamus.
D. T – The pineal body is found in the epithalamus.
E. F – The amygdala (amygdaloid nucleus) is considered to be part of the limbic system.

Further reading: Barr and Kiernan (1988; pp. 179–181)

1. 47

A. F – The abducens nucleus is situated in the pons.
B. T – The nucleus of the hypoglossal nerve (XII); the nucleus ambiguus, the origin of the cranial root of the accessory nerve (XI); the dorsal motor nucleus of the vagus (X) and the lateral, medial and inferior vestibular (VIII) are situated in the medulla.
C. T.
D. F – The facial nerve nucleus is located in the pons.
E. T.

Further reading: Brodal (1981; pp. 453–461, 472–473, 532–533; Barr and Kiernan (1988; pp. 92–103)

1.48 The following features are true of the resting neurone:

A. High intracellular concentration of potassium.
B. High intracellular concentration of sodium.
C. Low extracellular concentration of chloride.
D. High extracellular concentration of chloride.
E. The inside of the cell is positive compared with the fluids.

1.49 Neuropathological lesions characteristic of Wernicke's encephalopathy are seen in the following areas:

A. Mamillary bodies.
B. Corpus striatum.
C. Brainstem.
D. Hippocampus.
E. Structures adjacent to the third ventricle.

1.50 Characteristic neuropathological changes in Huntington's chorea include:

A. Atrophy of frontal and temporal lobes.
B. The presence of Lewy bodies.
C. Ventricular dilatation.
D. Atrophy of the striatum.
E. Thinning of the corpus callosum.

1.48

A. T – The resting nerve cell has a high intracellular concentration of potassium and a low intracellular concentration of sodium and chloride.
B. F.
C. F – In the extracellular fluid concentrations of sodium and chloride are high and of potassium low.
D. T.
E. F – The inside of the cell is strongly negative compared to the extracellular fluids.

Further reading: Gilman and Winans (1982)

1.49

A. T – Changes in Wernicke's encephalopathy are symmetrical and are seen in the area adjacent to the walls of the third ventricle, the periaqueductal region, the floor of the fourth ventricle, some thalamic nuclei, the mamillary bodies, the terminal portions of the fornices, the brainstem and the anterior lobe and superior vermis of the cerebellum.
B. F.
C. T.
D. F.
E. T.

Further reading: Lishman (1987; p. 495); Duchen and Jacobs (1992; pp. 813–817)

1.50

A. F – The brain is usually atrophied, particularly the frontal and parietal lobes.
B. F – These are seen in Parkinson's disease.
C. T.
D. T – The caudate and putamen are atrophied.
E. T.

Further reading: Lishman (1987; pp. 399–400); Oppenheimer and Esiri (1992; pp. 1002–1005)

Paper 2

2.1 Depersonalization experiences have been associated with the following:

A. Prolonged sleep deprivation.
B. Mania.
C. Sensory deprivation.
D. Temporal lobe epilepsy.
E. Catatonia.

2.2 Characteristic features of flight of ideas include:

A. Verbal stereotypy.
B. *Vorbeireden.*
C. Clang associations.
D. Perseveration.
E. Verbal associations.

2.3 Visual hallucinations:

A. Are not seen in blind or partially sighted people.
B. Can be associated with a homonymous hemianopia.
C. Can occur in narcolepsy.
D. Always have their origin in the occipital lobe.
E. Can occur in lesions of the diencephalon.

2.1

A. T – Transient depersonalization experiences are not uncommon in normal subjects in states of fatigue, after prolonged sleep deprivation, under conditions of sensory deprivation and under the influence of hallucinogenic drugs.
B. F – In psychiatric practice depersonalization is seen in depression, schizophrenia and hysteria.
C. T.
D. T.
E. F.

Further reading: Fish (1984; p. 58); Sedman (1970)

2.2

A. F – In verbal stereotypy the same word or phrase is used, regardless of the situation.
B. F – This is the German term for talking past the point. It is a result of loosened associations.
C. T.
D. F – This is the persistent and inappropriate repetition of the same thoughts.
E. T – In flight of ideas the associations of the train of thought can be determined by chance relationships, verbal associations of all kinds, clang associations, proverbs and clichés.

Further reading: Gelder *et al.* (1989; pp. 10–13)

2.3

A. F – In the syndrome of Bonnet visual hallucinations occur in the blind or partially sighted person. The hallucinations are of elementary or complex type, are of people or animals and are vividly coloured. They occur in the blind field.
B. T.
C. T – Hypnagogic hallucinations, often vivid and terrifying, accompany or precede sleep paralysis.
D. F – According to Penfield and Rasmussen, elementary hallucinations have their origin in lesions of the occipital cortex and complex ones in the temporal cortex.
E. T.

Further reading: Adams and Victor (1989; pp. 314, 368–369)

2.4 Characteristic features of the Ganser syndrome include:
A. Clear consciousness.
B. Consistent response to questions with approximate answers.
C. Pseudohallucinations.
D. An amnesia for the duration of the illness on recovery.
E. *Déjà vu* experiences.

2.5 Characteristic features of epileptic automatisms include:
A. Normal control of posture and tone.
B. Clear consciousness.
C. Complete recall for the period of the automatism.
D. They occur only after a seizure.
E. A normal EEG.

2.6 Characteristic features of pseudoseizures (psychogenic seizures or hysterical seizures) include:
A. Loss of consciousness.
B. Incontinence of urine.
C. Normal post 'seizure' EEG.
D. Cyanosis.
E. Classic generalized seizure.

2.4

A. F – Clouding of consciousness with disorientation is characteristic.
B. F – Approximate answers are interspersed with correct responses.
C. T – 'Hallucinations', when present, are usually visual and often elaborate. They are probably not true hallucinations but pseudohallucinations.
D. T.
E. F. The Ganser syndrome is classified as a dissociative disorder in *ICD-10*.

Further reading: Sims (1988; pp. 49–50); Enoch and Trethowan (1991; pp. 75–91); World Health Organization (1992)

2.5

A. T.
B. F – There is clouding of consciousness.
C. F – Amnesia for the period of the automatism is a constant feature.
D. F – Can also occur during the ictus.
E. F – Continuous electrical disturbance in the EEG (diffuse slow waves) is seen.

Further reading: Lishman (1987; pp. 221–222); Sims (1988; pp. 27–28)

2.6

A. F – There is no loss of consciousness, but the patient may be inaccessible.
B. F – Incontinence and tongue-biting are rare.
C. T – A normal EEG taken during or shortly after an attack provides firm evidence of a non-organic seizure.
D. F – Cyanosis and facial pallor are rarely seen.
E. F – Not a feature of pseudoseizures.

Further reading: Lishman (1987; pp. 259–261); Gelder *et al.* (1989; p. 205)

2.7 Overvalued ideas:

A. Are delusional in nature.
B. Are obsessional in nature.
C. Are usually associated with a very strong affect.
D. Often dominate the sufferer's life.
E. Have a good prognosis.

2.8 A patient with alcoholic hallucinosis:

A. Hears voices saying his or her thoughts out loud.
B. Hears voices saying simple words.
C. Hears voices giving a running commentary.
D. Only hears voices when abstinent from alcohol.
E. Shows evidence of thought disorder.

2.9 The following defence mechanisms are associated with Anna Freud:

A. Regression.
B. Projection.
C. Splitting.
D. Isolation.
E. Projective identification.

2.7 A. F – Wernicke (1900) established the concept of the overvalued idea and distinguished between it and obsessions and delusions.
B. F.
C. T – Jaspers believed that overvalued ideas were isolated notions associated with a strong affect and abnormal personality, and similar in quality to passionate, religious or ethical conviction.
D. T.
E. F – They carry a poor prognosis.

Further reading: McKenna (1984); Sims (1988; pp. 92–95)

2.8

A. F – Characteristic of schizophrenia.
B. T – Usually simple words or short sentences are heard. The patient is often spoken to in the second person.
C. F.
D. F – May also arise and occur while the patient continues to drink.
E. F.

Further reading: Glass (1989a, 1989b); Glass and Marshall (1991; pp. 152–162)

2.9

A. T – Regression is also associated with Sigmund Freud himself. In 1936, his daughter Anna described nine mechanisms of defence – regression, repression, reaction formation, isolation, undoing, projection, introjection, turning against the self and reversal.
B. T.
C. F – Melanie Klein emphasized the defences of splitting and projective identification.
D. T.
E. F.

Further reading: Brown and Pedder (1991; pp. 24–31)

2.10 The following statements concerning the treatment alliance are correct:

A. It can be called the working alliance.
B. It refers specifically to the relationship between the patient and the psychiatrist.
C. Trust is necessary for its development.
D. It can be reformulated as the patient's wish to get better.
E. The patient needs to be capable of tolerating a certain degree of frustration for it to develop.

2.11 Transference:

A. Is a term which was first used by Freud.
B. Was initially viewed as a clinical phenomenon which could act as an obstacle or resistance to analytic work.
C. Defines the process by which the patient displaces on to the analyst feelings and ideas which derive from previous figures in his or her life.
D. Can be used by the therapist to investigate the forgotten and repressed past.
E. Is directed towards the therapist in the therapeutic situation.

2.12 Gestalt therapy:

A. Was developed by Rogers.
B. Encourages transference.
C. Can be practised individually.
D. Includes the principle of here and now.
E. Involves the technique of 'rocking and rolling'.

2.10

A. T.
B. F – It can refer to the good relationship that any two people need to have in cooperating over a joint task.
C. T – The absence of basic trust is thought to account for the absence of a fully functional treatment alliance in certain psychotics and in others who have experienced severe emotional deprivation as children.
D. F – The patient's wish for recovery is a very unreliable basis for the treatment alliance. These patients very often break off treatment as soon as they achieve some symptomatic relief – 'flight into health'.
E. T.

Further reading: Sandler *et al.* (1970b)

2.11

A. T – In 1895.
B. T.
C. T.
D. T.
E. T.

Further reading: Sandler *et al.* (1970c); Brown and Pedder (1991; pp. 54–60)

2.12

A. F – Gestalt therapy was described by Fritz Perls.
B. F – In Gestalt therapy, transference is not encouraged. Instead, dramatization is used to explore and express fuller awareness of the self in the here and now.
C. T – Gestalt therapy can be practised individually, but is more usually practised in groups. It does not make use of group processes.
D. T – The principle of here and now is one of the basic rules of Gestalt therapy. Others include I and thou, It language, No gossiping, Dialogue, Making the rounds, Unfinished business, Exaggeration and Reversal.
E. F – 'Rocking and rolling' is one of the techniques used to facilitate 'basic encounter' in encounter groups.

Further reading: Brown and Pedder (1991; pp. 168, 171)

2.13 In the large group setting:
- A. A primary resistance is absenteeism.
- B. The emphasis is on psychotherapy.
- C. There should be several leaders.
- D. Features similar to the unconscious of psychoanalysis are displayed.
- E. There is little opportunity for dialogue.

2.14 In psychoanalytic theory, resistance:
- A. Is a psychological concept.
- B. Can provide information on the patient's mental functioning.
- C. Is synonymous with defence.
- D. May arise due to the threat posed by the analytic procedure.
- E. Is not an obstacle to treatment.

2.15 The following may be neuropsychiatric sequelae of subarachnoid haemorrhage:
- A. Depression.
- B. Anxiety.
- C. Persistent headache.
- D. Epilepsy.
- E. Organic mental symptoms.

2.13

A. T – Which can result finally in no group at all!
B. F – The emphasis is on sociocultural learning.
C. F – Conducting should be confined to one or two leaders. In a therapeutic community large group there are several members of staff present who might be called convenors, but amongst them is someone who is perceived as the leader.
D. T – The large group is primitive and unconscious on one hand, but potentially sophisticated on the other, because there is enormous opportunity to confront the unconscious with dialogue.
E. F.

Further reading: de Mare (1984)

2.14

A. F – It is a clinical rather than a psychological concept.
B. T – Emphasized by Anna Freud. It can reflect the type of conflict and the defences used.
C. F – Although resistance and defence are closely linked, they are not synonymous.
D. T.
E. F.

Further reading: Sandler *et al.* (1970e)

2.15

A. T – Common.
B. T – Occasionally this is severely disabling.
C. T.
D. T.
E. T.

Note: Follow-up studies of survivors of subarachoid haemorrhage report the following: paresis, epilepsy, persistent headache, organic mental symptoms, including memory impairment, anxiety and depression, and personality change (sometimes a deterioration in personality and sometimes an improvement).

Further reading: Lishman (1987; pp. 334–339)

2.16 In Huntington's chorea/Huntington's disease:
A. The onset is typically between the ages of 15 and 30.
B. Neurological signs may precede psychiatric symptoms.
C. Cognitive impairment occurs early in the course of the disease.
D. The initial diagnosis is retrospectively found to have been wrong in at least one-third of cases.
E. The chorea begins in the extremities in most cases.

2.17 The following are recognized features of Wernicke's encephalopathy:
A. Memory disorder.
B. Quadriplegia.
C. Pseudobulbar palsy.
D. Emotional abnormalities.
E. Peripheral neuropathy.

2.18 Characteristic features of functional stupor include:
A. Marked clouding of consciousness.
B. Aphasia.
C. Immobility.
D. Hyperreflexia.
E. Unresponsive.

2.16

A. F – The onset is typically between 25 and 60 with an average in the mid 40s.
B. T – Neurological signs precede psychiatric symptoms in just over half of the cases.
C. F – Cognitive impairment usually occurs late in the course and memory is often less affected than other aspects of cognitive impairment.
D. T.
E. T – The initial signs of involuntary movements are subtle, and mainly occur in the extremities.

Further reading: Martin (1984); Gelder *et al.* (1989; pp. 366–368); Lishman (1987; pp. 396–399)

2.17

A. T – This is frequently evident but hard to assess when confusion is present and is therefore often overlooked.
B. F.
C. F – Quadriplegia, pseudobulbar palsy and loss of pain sensation in the limbs and trunk are features of central pontine myelinosis, which is a demyelination, especially of the pyramidal tracts within the pons, and thought to be of nutritional aetiology.
D. T – These have been stressed in prisoner of war (POWs) patients, and include apprehension, anxiety, insomnia, fear of the dark, and later apathy, depression and emotional lability.
E. T – This has been described in treated POWs with Wernicke's encephalopathy.

Further reading: Lishman (1987; pp. 491–494, 500)

2.18

A. F – The patient appears to be fully conscious. When the eyes are open they are able to follow objects and when the eyes are closed they resist attempts to open them. The reflexes are normal and the resting posture is maintained.
B. F – Mute, not aphasic.
C. T.
D. F – Normal reflexes usually.
E. T.

Further reading: Lishman (1987; pp. 131–133); Gelder *et al.* (1989; p. 32)

2.19 Characteristic features of complex partial epilepsy include:
A. Impaired consciousness.
B. Aura.
C. Invariably leads to tonic-clonic phase.
D. Absences.
E. Often preceded by a simple partial seizure.

2.20 In Bleuler's view, the fundamental symptoms of schizophrenia included:
A. Disturbances of associations.
B. Autism.
C. Catatonia.
D. Hallucinations.
E. Delusions.

2.21 The following are examples of loosening of associations seen in schizophrenia:
A. Neologisms.
B. Word salad.
C. Punning.
D. Metonyms.
E. Parapraxes.

2.19

A. T.
B. T – This is typically an epigastric aura, a sensation of churning felt in the stomach and spreading towards the neck.
C. F – A generalized seizure may occur secondary to a complex partial seizure, but it is not feature of a complex partial seizure. In a complex partial seizure the individual loses touch with the surroundings and may show automatisms.
D. F – An absence seizure starts without an aura and ends abruptly.
E. T.

Further reading: Gelder *et al.* (1989; pp. 389–392)

2.20

A. T
B. T.
C. F.
D. F.
E. F.

Note: Bleuler (1857–1959) coined the term schizophrenia. He thought that the fundamental symptoms were disturbances of associations, changes in emotional reactions, tendency to prefer fantasy to reality and autism. His accessory symptoms included hallucinations, delusions, catatonia and abnormal behaviour.

Further reading: Gelder *et al.* (1989; pp. 277–278)

2.21

A. T.
B. T.
C. F – Seen in mania.
D. T – This is the use of ordinary words in unusual ways.
E. F – Paraphrasias are examples of loosening of associations seen in schizophrenia; parapraxes are slips of the tongue.

Further reading: Gelder *et al.* (1989; p. 271)

2.22 Characteristic features of classic tardive dyskinesia in schizophrenia include:
- A. A late onset.
- B. Choreoathetoid movements of lips, tongue and mouth.
- C. When extremities are involved, hands are more commonly affected than the feet.
- D. The rabbit syndrome.
- E. Subjective feeling of restlessness or uneasiness.

2.23 Positive symptoms of schizophrenia include:
- A. Hallucinations.
- B. Flat affect.
- C. Delusions.
- D. Poverty of speech.
- E. Avolition.

2.22

A. T.
B. T.
C. T.
D. F – The rabbit syndrome is another late onset movement disorder that can be confused with tardive dyskinesia. It involves rapid, fine rhythmic movements of the mouth that resemble the chewing movements of rabbits. Unlike TD, it improves with anticholinergics.
E. F – This is the definition of akathisia, which can also occur in a tardive form. Barnes and Braude (1985) report that tardive dyskinesia can sometimes include akathisia, though this is not the characteristic picture.

Further reading: Barnes and Braude (1985); Hanson (1988)

2.23

A. T – All operationalized definitions include delusions and hallucinations.
B. F – All operationalized definitions of negative symptoms include flat affect and poverty of speech.
C. T.
D. F.
E. F – Most operationalized definitions include avolition, anhedonia, apathy and abulia in the category of negative symptoms.

Note: Thought disorder, bizarre behaviour and inappropriate affect are variably classified as positive or negative. It is now suggested that they constitute a third factor that is orthogonal to the positive–negative distinction.

Further reading: McGlashen and Fenton (1992)

2.24 The following are common important features of chronic (defect state) schizophrenia:
A. Cognitive impairment.
B. Thought insertion.
C. Depression.
D. Delusional perception.
E. Emotional blunting.

2.25 The following movement disorders occur in schizophrenia:
A. Stereotypy.
B. Logoclonia.
C. Ambitendence.
D. Echopraxia.
E. Choreiform movements.

2.24

A. T.
B. F – Thought insertion is more commonly a feature of the acute illness, although it may persist.
C. T – Depression is a common feature of chronic schizophrenia, although it has also been described in the immediate post-psychotic period. Approximately 10% of schizophrenics die by suicide, usually in the early years of their illness.
D. F.
E. T – Apathy and emotional blunting are permanent changes in the personality which handicap the chronic schizophrenic. Other prominent features include reduced drive, social withdrawal, emotional blunting and recurrent psychotic episodes.

Further reading: Kendall (1993; pp. 379–426)

2.25

A. T – A repeated movement which does not appear to be goal-directed, e.g. rocking forwards or backwards.
B. F – This describes the spastic repetition of syllables that occurs in Parkinson's disease.
C. T – A form of ambivalence. The patient starts to make a movement, but before completing it, starts the opposite movement.
D. T – This is when the patient imitates the interviewer's every action, despite having been asked not to.
E. T – Choreiform movements are seen in tardive dyskinesia, which may occur in schizophrenics who have never received any neuroleptic drugs.

Further reading: Manschreck *et al.* (1982); Sims (1988; pp. 128, 273–278); Gelder *et al.* (1989; p. 273)

2.26 The following are typical features of *ICD-10* post-traumatic stress disorder (PTSD):

A. It arises within 6 months of a traumatic event of exceptional severity.
B. Avoidance of activities and situations reminiscent of the trauma.
C. Flashbacks.
D. Hypervigilance.
E. Insomnia.

2.27 Biological symptoms of depression can include:

A. Weight loss.
B. Diurnal variation of mood.
C. Constipation.
D. Loss of libido.
E. Amenorrhoea.

2.28 The following are increased in depressed patients:

A. Prolactin response to infusions of L-tryptophan.
B. Prolactin response to oral fenfluramine.
C. Postmortem brain dopamine concentrations.
D. Cerebrospinal fluid (CSF) 5-hydroxyindoleacetic acid (5-HIAA).
E. Growth hormone response to clonidine.

2.26

A. T.
B. T.
C. T – These are episodes of repeated reliving of the trauma in intrusive memories and occur against the persisting background of a sense of numbness and emotional blunting, detachment from other people, unresponsiveness to surroundings, anhedonia and avoidance of activities and situations reminiscent of the trauma.
D. T.
E. T.

Further reading: World Health Organization (1992)

2.27

A. T.
B. T.
C. T.
D. T.
E. T.

Note: Also, sleep disturbance with early morning wakening and loss of appetite.

Further reading: Gelder *et al.* (1989; pp. 219–220)

2.28

A. F – Reduced. L-Tryptophan is a precursor of 5-HT and infusion enhances 5-HT function.
B. F.
C. F – No significant changes have been reported in post-mortem brains of depressed patients.
D. F – On balance, evidence is found for reduced concentrations.
E. F – Several studies have shown a reduced GH response to clonidine in depressed patients, suggesting a defect in postsynaptic noradrenergic receptors.

Further reading: Gelder *et al.* (1989; pp. 246–250)

2.29 The following are true of unipolar depressive disorders:
A. They begin on average in the mid 20s.
B. They are commoner in women.
C. They are more frequent in higher social classes.
D. They breed true.
E. They are more likely to become chronic than bipolar disorders.

2.30 Characteristic features of Cotard's syndrome include:
A. Delusion of negation.
B. Commoner in women.
C. Insidious onset.
D. Onset in the 20s.
E. Association with a depressive illness.

2.31 The maternity blues:
A. Occur in about 50–70% of recently delivered women.
B. Do not occur after home births.
C. Are associated with obstetric complications.
D. Are more likely to occur in women who have experienced depressive symptoms in late pregnancy.
E. Typically reach their peak on the third or fourth postpartum day.

2.29

A. F – Bipolar disorders have an onset in the mid 20s. Unipolar states have an onset in the mid 30s.
B. T – There is a female prepondrance in unipolar disorders. The sex ratio in bipolar states is approximately equal.
C. F – But bipolar disorders are.
D. T.
E. T – Adverse factors include being female, high familial loading and physical ill health and disability in the elderly.

Further reading: Gelder *et al.* (1989; pp. 235–236); Weller (1992; pp. 533–534)

2.30

A. T – Sometimes called by the French name *délire de négation.*
B. T.
C. F – The onset is typically acute.
D. F – Usually presents in late middle life.
E. T – Although it can occur in association with other psychotic states, e.g. acute schizophrenia and organic psychosyndromes.

Further reading: Enoch and Trethowan (1991; pp. 162–183)

2.31

A. T – And some reports have found an increased incidence in primiparous women.
B. F – The incidence in home-birth studies is about 60–70%, thus it is unlikely that hospitalization plays a causal role.
C. F – Apart from a possible association with the length of labour, no obstetric variable has been found to correlate with the maternity blues.
D. T – And in women with a history of premenstrual tension.
E. T – Although weeping and depression may persist for several weeks.

Note: The term maternity blues fails to convey that many women are also elated at this time.

Further reading: Stein (1982; pp. 119–154)

2.32 Characteristic features of schizoid personality disorder (*DSM-IV/ICD-10*) include:

A. A strong association with schizophrenia.
B. Lack of emotional warmth.
C. A predilection for solitary activities.
D. Excessive social anxiety.
E. Paranoid ideation.

2.33 Schizophrenia spectrum disorders include:

A. Schizotypal personality disorder.
B. Obsessive-compulsive personality disorder.
C. Paranoid personality disorder.
D. Schizoid personality disorder.
E. Narcissistic personality disorder.

2.34 The following are true of adjustment disorders (*ICD-10*):

A. They are out of proportion to the severity of the stressful experience.
B. They are closely associated in time and content to the stressor.
C. They occur in people previously free of medical disorder.
D. Symptoms can include aggressive behaviour.
E. They are chronic disorders.

2.32

A. F – The association is weak.
B. T.
C. T.
D. F – Excessive social anxiety is seen in schizotypal personality disorder.
E. F.

Further reading: American Psychiatric Association (1994); World Health Organization (1992)

2.33

A. T – The concept of schizophrenia spectrum is gaining recognition. The disorders most commonly placed within this spectrum are schizotypal personality disorder, schizoid personality disorder, schizoaffective disorder, schizophreniform disorder and paranoid personality disorder. Delusional disorders, brief reactive psychoses and psychogenic psychoses may also lie within the spectrum.
B. F.
C. T.
D. T.
E. F.

Further reading: Wigider *et al.* (1988)

2.34

A. F – The disorder is understandable and in proportion to the severity of the stressful experience.
B. T – These disorders follow life changes or stressful life events and usually develop within 1 month of the event in question.
C. T.
D. T – Symptoms usually include depressed mood, anxiety, worry and irritability. Aggressive behaviour has also been described.
E. F – Adjustment disorders are typically mild or transient disorders which last longer than acute reactions; the symptoms are varied, are generally reversible and last a few months.

Further reading: Freeman (1993; p. 519); Gelder *et al.* (1989; pp. 163–164); World Health Organization (1992)

2.35 Social phobia:

A. Is equally frequent in men and women.
B. Usually begins in childhood.
C. Is associated with alcohol abuse.
D. Has an insidious onset.
E. Is best treated by anxiolytic drugs.

2.36 The following are characteristics of obsessional thoughts:

A. They are the patient's own thoughts.
B. They are recognized as being senseless.
C. They are a form of thought disorder.
D. They can reach delusional intensity.
E. They are generally about matters which the patient finds distressing.

2.35

A. T – Unlike most other phobias.
B. F – Usually begins between the ages of 17 and 30 years.
C. T – Social phobics more commonly abuse alcohol than other phobics. Abuse of anxiolytic drugs is also common. Social phobia is also associated with depression.
D. F – Typically has a recognizable onset. The first episode is usually remembered, and has occurred without a precipitant, in a public place.
E. F – Cognitive behavioural therapy is the treatment of choice. Anxiolytic drugs are best used briefly to diminish symptoms until cognitive behavioural therapy has effect.

Further reading: Liebowitz *et al.* (1985); Gelder *et al.* (1989; pp. 185–186); Freeman (1993; pp. 501–502)

2.36

A. T – Obsessional thoughts are repetitive, intrusive ideas which are always recognized by the subject as his or her own.
B. T – They are experienced as being absurd and senseless.
C. F – See A.
D. F – They are usually concerned with unacceptable ideas about violence, sex and obscenity.
E. T.

Further reading: Marks (1987; pp. 431–432); Gelder *et al.* (1989; pp. 22–23); Freeman (1993; pp. 504–510)

2.37 The differential diagnosis of generalized anxiety disorder (GAD) includes:

A. Myasthenia gravis.
B. Thyrotoxicosis.
C. Neurasthenia.
D. Alcohol dependence.
E. Hypoglycaemia.

2.38 Dopamine is particularly localized in the following brain areas:

A. Locus coeruleus.
B. Ventromedial tegmental area.
C. Nigrostriatal area.
D. Nucleus basalis of Meynert.
E. Midbrain raphe nuclei.

2.37

A. F – This presents with weakness and fatigue.
B. T – Patients presenting with GAD should be assessed clinically for features of thyroid disease.
C. T – The core symptoms of this disorder are excessive fatigue and lethargy, but symptoms of anxiety and depression also occur.
D. T – Alcohol-dependent individuals typically complain of anxiety in the early morning, when their blood alcohol levels have dropped and they are experiencing withdrawal symptoms.
E. T – Hypoglycaemia and phaeochromocytoma should be considered when symptoms are episodic.

Note: Other physical problems to be ruled out include parathyroid disease and cardiac conditions (mitral valve prolapse, paroxysmal atrial tachycardia).

Further reading: American Psychiatric Association (1994); Gelder *et al.* (1989, pp. 178–179); World Health Organization (1992); Freeman (1993; pp. 497–500)

2.38

A. F – Noradrenaline-containing cell bodies are located here.
B. T.
C. T.
D. F – Cholinergic cell bodies are located here.
E. F – Serotoninergic cell bodies are located here.

Further reading: Shanks (1984; p. 21); Silverstone and Turner (1988; pp. 10–15)

2.39 Chlorpromazine:
A. Is a piperidine phenothiazine.
B. Has marked antimuscarinic effects.
C. Blocks postsynaptic dopamine receptors.
D. Causes increased turnover of dopamine.
E. Has a plasma half-life of some 6 hours.

2.40 The following foods should be avoided on MAOIs:
A. Eggs.
B. Broad bean pods.
C. Beer.
D. Snails.
E. Large quantities of chocolate.

2.39

A. F – Chlorpromazine is a phenothiazine with an aliphatic side chain. Thioridazine has a piperidine side chain. Fluphenazine has a piperazine side chain.

B. F – Chlorpromazine has moderate antimuscarinic side-effects. Thioridazine has more marked antimuscarinic side-effects.

C. T.

D. T – After the postsynaptic dopamine receptors have been blocked, there is a feedback mechanism which causes an increased production and turnover of dopamine, with a corresponding increase in its metabolites.

E. T – However, it can remain bound for very long periods and metabolites may continue to be excreted for up to 6 months after the patient has stopped taking it.

Further reading: Silverstone and Turner (1988; pp. 110–115); *British National Formulary* (1994; p. 153)

2.40

A. F – Eggs have not been implicated as having toxic effects with MAOIs.

B. T – Hypertensive crisis is a serious toxic effect of MAO inhibitors related to ingestion of foods containing tyramine and other substances. The most dangerous foods are mature cheeses and yeast products used as food supplements. Other foods include beer, wine, pickled herring, snails, game, chicken liver, yeast and yeast extracts; also large quantities of coffee, citrus fruits, and chocolate or cream and their products. Food which may be 'going off' (meat, fish, poultry or offal) is also implicated.

C. T.

D. T.

E. T.

Further reading: Silverstone and Turner (1988; p. 164); Baldessarini (1990; pp. 414–418)

2.41 The following are recognized side-effects of MAOIs:

A. Suppressed rapid eye movement (REM) sleep.
B. Peripheral neuropathy.
C. Hypotension.
D. Hypertension.
E. Arthritis.

2.42 Recognized features of tricyclic antidepressants include:

A. Lipophilic.
B. Cannot be given intramuscularly.
C. Strongly bound to plasma proteins.
D. Are metabolized more slowly in children.
E. Tertiary amines preferentially block uptake of noradrenaline.

2.43 Carbamazepine is recognized to be an effective treatment in the following conditions:

A. Acute mania.
B. Obsessive-compulsive disorder.
C. Status epilepticus.
D. Prophylaxis of bipolar affective disorder.
E. Defect state schizophrenia.

2.41

A. T – MAOIs are highly effective suppressors of REM sleep, and this effect has been used therapeutically in the treatment of narcolepsy.
B. T – Peripheral neuropathy following MAOI use may be related to pyridoxine deficiency.
C. T.
D. T.
E. F – Not described, though a recognized side-effect of mianserin.

Further reading: Baldessarini (1990; pp. 414–418); *British National Formulary* (1994; pp. 167–168)

2.42

A. T.
B. F.
C. T.
D. F – Are metabolized more rapidly in children and more slowly in patients over 60.
E. F – They preferentially block the uptake of 5-HT.

Further reading: Baldessarini (1990; pp. 405–414)

2.43

A. T – However, it lacks the initial sedative properties of many neuroleptics and the need for a gradual elevation in dosage makes its use less convenient.
B. F – Little response reported in the literature.
C. F – Diazepam intravenously or rectally is the recognized treatment.
D. T – Well-recognized.
E. F – Overactivity, aggression and poor impulse control in a variety of psychiatric diagnoses, including schizophrenia, *may* improve with carbamazepine, but carbamazepine on its own is not a consistently effective treatment.

Further reading: Silverstone and Turner (1988; pp. 160, 170–171); Elphick (1989)

2.44 The following drugs are excreted in breast milk:
A. Lithium carbonate.
B. Amitriptyline.
C. Sulpiride.
D. Carbamazepine.
E. Diazepam.

2.45 Components of the basal ganglia include:
A. Claustrum.
B. Caudate nucleus.
C. Cingulate gyrus.
D. Thalamus.
E. Lentiform (lenticular) nucleus.

2.46 The following are features of the cerebellum:
A. It receives afferents from the proprioceptor organs of the body.
B. It contains Purkinje cells.
C. It contains Golgi cells.
D. Lesions produce contralateral effects.
E. It obtains blood supply from the middle cerebral artery.

2.44

A. T – Good control of maternal plasma concentrations minimizes risk of intoxication.
B. T – The amount excreted is too small to be harmful.
C. T – A significant amount of sulpiride is excreted in breast milk and is thus best avoided.
D. T – The amount is too small to be harmful.
E. T – Repeated doses should be avoided. Lethargy and weight loss may occur in infant.

Further reading: *British National Formulary* (1994; pp. 551–556)

2.45

A. T – The claustrum is usually included.
B. T – The caudate nucleus and the lentiform nucleus (putamen and globus pallidus) make up the main mass of the basal ganglia.
C. F – The cingulate gyrus is part of the limbic lobe.
D. F.
E. T.

Further reading: Brodal (1981; p. 211); Barr and Kiernan (1988; pp. 344–345)

2.46

A. T – Although it receives a large number of proprioceptive afferents, conscious perception does not occur in the cerebellum.
B. T – The cerebellum consists of three layers – the molecular, Purkinje and granular cell layers. Purkinje cell bodies are located in the Purkinje cell layer and Golgi type II cells in the granular cell layer.
C. T.
D. F – Cerebellar lesions produce ipsilateral effects.
E. F.

Further reading: Barr and Kiernan (1988; pp. 160–177)

2.47 Recognized features of motor neurone disease include:
A. Dysphasia.
B. Muscle fasciculation.
C. Incontinence of urine.
D. Exaggerated tendon reflexes.
E. Muscle atrophy.

2.48 Characteristic neuropathological features of Alzheimer's disease include:
A. Severe parieto-occipital atrophy.
B. Neuronal degeneration.
C. Senile plaques in white matter.
D. Neurofibrillary tangles.
E. Glial proliferation.

2.49 The following neuropathological features are recognized in Korsakoff's psychosis:
A. Marked atrophy of the caudate nuclei.
B. Lesions in the dorsomedial nucleus of the thalamus.
C. Cortical atrophy.
D. Cerebellar lesions.
E. Ventricular dilatation.

2.47

A. F – Dysarthria and dysphagia occur.
B. T – Muscle wasting and fasciculation often occur in the disease.
C. F – The sphincters are not usually affected, though a slight precipitancy and difficulty of micturition are not uncommon.
D. T.
E. T.

Further reading: Barr and Kiernan (1988; pp. 341–342)

2.48

A. F – Cortical atrophy is generalized but affects the fronto-temporal lobes more severely than the parieto-occipital region.
B. T – Neuronal degeneration, especially of the outer three cortical layers.
C. F – Senile plaques are not seen in the white matter in Alzheimer's. They are scattered densely throughout the cortex. The subcortical grey matter is less severely affected.
D. T.
E. T.

Further reading: Lishman (1987; pp. 380–383); Tomlinson (1992; pp. 1317–1341)

2.49

A. F – This is a feature of Huntington's chorea.
B. T – Responsible for the memory disorder.
C. T.
D. T – Degeneration of all layers of the cortex, particularly of the Purkinje cells; usually confined to the superior part of the vermis.
E. T.

Further reading: Lishman (1987; p. 497); Duchen and Jacobs (1992; pp. 813–817)

2.50 Characteristic pathological features of Pick's disease include:

A. Cerebellar atrophy.
B. The presence of balloon cells.
C. Atrophy of the basal ganglia.
D. Preservation of myelin in white matter of affected lobes.
E. The presence of Pick bodies.

2.50

A. F – There is generalized atrophy, involving mainly the frontal and temporal lobes. The cerebellum is usually spared.
B. T – These are characteristic cells.
C. T – The basal ganglia and thalamus show atrophy.
D. F – Loss of myelin in white matter of affected lobes is usually considerable.
E. T – Affected neurons are swollen, with loss of Nissl substance and irregular shaped argentophilic inclusions (Pick bodies).

Further reading: Lishman (1987; pp. 392–393); Tomlinson (1992; pp. 1354–1361)

Paper 3

3.1 Depersonalization is:

A. A delusion.
B. A subjective experience.
C. Commonly felt to be an unpleasant experience.
D. A term used to describe a peculiar change in the awareness of the self in which the individual feels as if he or she is unreal.
E. A term used to describe a situation in which an individual denies that he or she exists or is alive.

3.2 The following are true of hallucinations:

A. They are restricted to the mentally ill.
B. Autoscopy is a special type of hallucination.
C. Extracampine hallucinations are located outside the perceptual field.
D. They are transformations of perceptions.
E. They are experienced as originating within the mind.

3.1

A. F – Insight is retained.
B. T.
C. T – Depersonalization experiences are often unpleasant experiences, and at times very distressing.
D. T – Sedman's definition.
E. F – This is a nihilistic delusion.

Further reading: Ackner (1954); Sedman (1970)

3.2

A. F.
B. T – This is a strange experience in which the subject sees himself projected into external space.
C. T – Hallucinations occurring outside the limits of the sensory field (i.e. outside the visual field or beyond the range of audibility).
D. F – Esquirol (1838) differentiated illusions from hallucinations. He described illusions as transformations of perceptions and hallucinations as perceptions without an object.
E. F – They are experienced as originating in the outside world.

Further reading: Sims (1988; pp. 65–69; 155–156); Gelder *et al.* (1989; pp. 6–10)

3.3 The following are examples of visual hallucinations:

A. Positive scotomata.
B. Fortification spectra.
C. After-image.
D. *Lilliputian* hallucinations.
E. Metamorphopsia.

3.4 Features more suggestive of a chronic, rather than an acute, organic reaction include:

A. Disorientation.
B. Fluctuation in consciousness.
C. Prominent illusions and visual hallucinations.
D. Pyrexia.
E. Neck stiffness.

3.3

A. T – These are simple percepts which obliterate part of the visual field, e.g. flashes and stars seen after a blow on the head.
B. T – These are scintillating luminous zigzag shapes perceived during a migraine attack (teichopsia) and thought to be due to ischaemia of nerve cells in the occipital lobe.
C. T – After-images are perceived in the field of vision when we have been looking at a bright light and then look away. Because they no longer correspond to any object in our central field of vision, they are therefore hallucinations. They are short-lived.
D. T – In delirium tremens visual hallucinations are frequently *Lilliputian* in size.
E. F – A visual illusion.

Further reading: Kräupl-Taylor (1979; pp. 104–108); Adams and Victor (1989; p. 204)

3.4

A. F – Occurs in both, although the quality is different.
B. F – True for acute organic reaction.
C. F – Seen in acute organic reactions.
D. F – This may indicate an infection causing an acute organic reaction.
E. F – This may indicate subarachnoid haemorrhage or meningitis, implying an acute organic reaction.

Further reading: Lishman (1987; pp. 126–133)

3.5 Paranoid delusions characteristically include:

A. Persecutory delusions.
B. Delusions of reference.
C. Hypochondriacal delusions.
D. Erotic delusions.
E. Depressive delusions.

3.6 The following features are commoner in schizophrenia-like psychoses of epilepsy when compared with typical schizophrenia:

A. A warm effect.
B. Positive family history of schizophrenia.
C. Auditory hallucinations.
D. Visual hallucinations.
E. Personality deterioration.

3.5

A. T – Persecutory delusions are the most characteristic form of paranoid delusions. Paranoid delusions occur in schizophrenia especially, but also in organic and depressive psychoses. They include delusions of persecution, delusions of reference, delusions of jealousy, litigious delusions, erotic delusions and occasionally grandiose delusions.
B. T – A patient with delusions of reference finds ego-involved meaning in everything that happens around him or her.
C. F – Hypochondriacal delusions occupy an uncertain position amongst delusional categories. Strictly defined, they include delusions occurring in organically determined disorders of body image, in states of clouded consciousness and in schizophrenia and depression.
D. T.
E. F – These have their basis in psychotic convictions of personal failure (e.g. delusions of guilt and unworthiness).

Further reading: Kräupl-Taylor (1979; pp. 130–135)

3.6

A. T.
B. F – Typically no family history.
C. F.
D. T – Visual hallucinations, often with a mystical content, are more common in schizophrenia-like psychoses of epilepsy than schizophrenia.
E. F – The progress of the disorder is more benign, with less personality and social deterioration.

Further reading: Fenton (1993; pp. 343–357)

3.7 Characteristic features of the Kleine–Levin syndrome include:

A. Periodic somnolence.
B. Periodic anorexia.
C. Usually occurs in young women.
D. Mental abnormalities during attacks include visual and auditory hallucinations.
E. The patient is normal between attacks.

3.8 The following symptoms indicate a diagnosis of hyperthyroidism rather than anxiety neurosis:

A. Tachycardia.
B. Preference for cold.
C. Increased appetite.
D. Palpitations.
E. Fine finger tremor.

3.7

A. T – The patient sleeps excessively by day and night during an attack. When awake, he is extremely hungry and eats voraciously. During attacks patients can be roused from daytime sleep, but then tend to be irritable and aggressive. Attacks last for several days to several weeks, with an average frequency of two per year.
B. F – See above.
C. F – Usually occurs in young men with an onset in early adolescence. Occasional cases occur in women, with an onset in middle age.
D. T.
E. T.

Further reading: Lishman (1987; pp. 628–629); Sims (1988; pp. 34–35)

3.8

A. F – Both show tachycardia, but in hyperthyroidism the sleeping heart rate is over 90 beats per minute.
B. T – Sensitivity to heat and preference for cold are good discriminating symptoms.
C. T – Increased appetite with weight loss indicate hyperthyroidism. Weight loss can occur in anxiety neurosis, due to reduced appetite.
D. F – Both show palpitations.
E. F – Occurs in both.

Further reading: Lishman (1987; p. 431)

3.9 The following associations are correct:

A. Neo-Freudians: Fromm.
B. Attachment behaviour: Bowlby.
C. Object relations: Lorenz.
D. Aggression: Jung.
E. Primal scream: Reich.

3.10 The following statements about Client-Centred Psychotherapy are correct:

A. It provides an enabling relationship.
B. It fosters regression.
C. It is non-directive.
D. Analysis of transference phenomena is an integral part of the therapy.
E. Effective therapists must be passive.

3.9

A. T – Fromm, Horney, Sullivan and Erikson were neo-Freudians.
B. T – Bowlby considered attachment as an important primary drive in higher primates, reaching a peak in humans between the ages of 9 months and 3 years.
C. F – Object relations theorists included Fairbairn, Guntrip, Winnicott and Balint. They suggested that the primary motivational drive in humans is to seek relationships with others. Konrad Lorenz was an ethologist.
D. F – Associated with Adler.
E. F – *The Primal Scream* is a book by Arthur Janov. Wilhelm Reich was one of the original followers of Freud.

Further reading: Brown and Pedder (1991; pp. 37–46, 176)

3.10

A. T – To allow the individual to realize his or her capacity for growth and self-realization.
B. F – Classical psychoanalysis fosters regression, transference of feeling towards the analyst and recollection of forgotten memories. In Client-Centred Psychotherapy the therapist's activity is mainly reflecting what the client says and paraphrasing the words.
C. T – The Client-Centred Psychotherapy of Carl Rogers has been a major influence in the field of non-directive counselling.
D. F – Rogerian therapists do not confront defences or interpret unconscious processes such as transference phenomena.
E. F – Effective therapists have three characteristics: accurate empathy, non-possessive warmth and genuineness.

Further reading: Brown and Pedder (1991; pp. 94–95)

3.11 The following are prerequisites for insight-oriented psychotherapy:

A. Verbal fluency.
B. Above average intelligence.
C. A degree of introspectiveness.
D. Adequate ego strength.
E. Assertiveness.

3.12 In psychoanalytic theory, the ego:

A. Is concerned with external reality.
B. Is not involved with defence mechanisms.
C. Is largely suspended in sleep.
D. Is not impaired in the acute psychotic disorders.
E. Is concerned with object relations.

3.13 Countertransference:

A. Was initially seen by Freud to be an obstacle to treatment.
B. Refers to the specific emotional responses aroused in the analyst by the specific qualities of the patient.
C. Can be a useful therapeutic tool.
D. Describes the analyst's unresolved conflicts and problems transferred on to the patient.
E. Can be extended outside the psychoanalytic treatment.

3.11

A. T.
B. F – Average intelligence is adequate.
C. T – A degree of introspectiveness is important, otherwise patients find it hard to reflect and think about their feelings.
D. T.
E. F.

Further reading: Brown and Pedder (1991; pp. 183–186)

3.12

A. T – Concerned with rational thinking, external perception and voluntary motor action.
B. F – Brings the defence mechanisms into action.
C. T – Ego functions are relaxed during sleep and fatigue and under the influence of drugs and alcohol.
D. F.
E. T – The ego is at the centre of object relations, both as they are represented in our inner world and in the outer world.

Further reading: Brown and Pedder (1991; p. 47)

3.13

A. T.
B. T – The countertransference has two elements: the analyst's own unresolved conflicts and problems transferred on to the patient and the specific emotional response giving information about the patient's unconscious processes.
C. T – Evaluation of the countertransference may enable the therapist to engage with the patient more deeply and effectively.
D. T.
E. T – And is a useful element in any doctor–patient or therapist–patient relationship.

Further reading: Sandler *et al.* (1970d); Brown and Pedder (1991; pp. 61–64)

3.14 In psychoanalytic theory, acting out:

A. Describes certain behavioural phenomena which arise during the course of an analysis which are a consequence of that treatment.
B. Has unconscious determinants.
C. Only occurs within the analytic situation.
D. Was referred to by Freud as a way of remembering.
E. Is viewed exclusively as a form of resistance.

3.15 In head injury, the duration of retrograde amnesia is closely correlated with:

A. Psychiatric disability.
B. Change of personality after head injury.
C. Generalized intellectual impairment.
D. Dysphasia.
E. Persistent deficits in memory.

3.16 Characteristic causes of the amnesic (Wernicke–Korsakoff) syndrome include:

A. Gastric carcinoma.
B. Hyperemesis gravidarum.
C. Multiple sclerosis.
D. Guillain–Barré syndrome.
E. Carbon monoxide poisoning.

3.14

A. T – This describes one of the main ways in which the concept has been used. It has also been used to describe habitual modes of action and behaviour which are related to the individual rather than to the treatment process.
B. T.
C. F.
D. T – Within the treatment situation the patient produces actions as substitutes for forgotten and repressed memories.
E. F – It must also be evaluated as a possible first source of new material emerging from unconscious drives.

Further reading: Sandler *et al.* (1970f)

3.15

A. F.
B. F.
C. F.
D. F.
E. F.

Note: These are all correlated with the duration of post-traumatic amnesia (PTA), the time between the injury and the resumption of normal continuous memory. Retrograde amnesia (RA) is the time between the injury and the last memory recalled before the injury and is not a good predictor of outcome.

Further reading: Gelder *et al.* (1989; pp. 369–372)

3.16

A. T – Acts via thiamine deficiency.
B. T – But rarely seen today.
C. F.
D. F – Guillain–Barré syndrome is an idiopathic or postinfectious polyneuropathy that does not involve any memory disturbance.
E. T.

Further reading: Gelder *et al.* (1989; pp. 355–356)

3.17 The following features are more suggestive of Pick's disease than Alzheimer's disease:

A. Incontinence occurring early in the course of the illness.
B. Marked memory disturbance at the onset.
C. Marked gait disturbance.
D. Apraxia and agnosia.
E. Normal EEG.

3.18 Psychiatric disorders characteristically associated with hypothyroidism include:

A. Organic psychosis.
B. Dementia.
C. Mania.
D. Depressive psychosis.
E. Capgras syndrome.

3.19 In patients with narcolepsy:

A. Nocturnal sleep is normal.
B. The routine EEG shows no abnormalities.
C. There may be a positive family history.
D. Daytime sleep attacks may be accompanied by REM sleep.
E. There is usually evidence of organic brain disease when narcolepsy and cataplexy are found together.

3.17

A. T.
B. F – Characteristic of Alzheimer's disease.
C. F – Less common in Pick's disease, as are extrapyramidal features.
D. F – These sometimes appear but are more common in Alzheimer's disease.
E. T – The EEG is normal, even in the presence of moderately advanced dementia.

Further reading: Lishman (1987; pp. 391–393)

3.18

A. T – This is the commonest syndrome – either acute or subacute, with delirium, florid delusions and hallucinations, mental confusion and impaired consciousness.
B. T – This progresses insidiously and may have reached an advanced degree by the time the diagnosis is made.
C. F – Not typically seen with hypothyroidism, but has been described in association with hyperthyroidism.
D. T – Both depressive and schizophrenic psychoses occur and may be accompanied by organic mental features.
E. F.

Further reading: Lishman (1987; pp. 432–436)

3.19

A. F – Is is disrupted.
B. T – The routine EEG shows no abnormalities. (The nocturnal sleep of narcoleptics is abnormal, with unusually early onset of REM sleep. Daytime sleep attacks also consist of REM-type sleep).
C. T – In approximately one-third of patients there is a positive family history. In occasional families the disorder has been shown to be transmitted as an autosomal dominant. Almost all cases have the human leukocyte antigen (HLA) type DR2, compared with one-quarter of the general population (chromosome 6).
D. T.
E. F.

Further reading: Parkes JD (1985; pp. 275–314); Lishman (1987; pp. 617–626); Gelder *et al.* (1989; pp. 401–402)

3.20 The following names are associated with the correct terms:
- A. Griesinger: unitary psychosis.
- B. Leonhard: schizophreniform.
- C. Kahlbaum: catatonia.
- D. Kraepelin: hebephrenia.
- E. Falret: *Démence précoce*.

3.21 Catatonic symptoms include:
- A. Sopor.
- B. Excitement.
- C. Cataplexy.
- D. *Mitgehen*.
- E. Confabulation.

3.22 Tardive dyskinesia:
- A. Is commoner in men.
- B. Is commoner in the elderly.
- C. Is commoner in patients who have diffuse brain pathology.
- D. May be aggravated by stopping antipsychotic drugs.
- E. Is associated with the duration of antipsychotic drug treatment.

3.20

A. T – Griesinger believed that all psychoses were different expressions of one common disease (*Einheitpsychose*).
B. F – Leonhard distinguished schizophrenia from 'cycloid' psychoses, which he described as a group of non-affective psychoses of good outcome.
C. T – Kahlbaum described this syndrome in 1863.
D. F – Hecker wrote an account of hebephrenia in 1871; Kraepelin (1855–1926) proposed dementia praecox and manic-depressive psychosis.
E. F – Falret described *folie circulaire* and Morel described *démence précoce*.

Further reading: Fish (1984; pp. 10–12); Gelder *et al.* (1989; pp. 276–279)

3.21

A. F – Sopor is a state of marked drowsiness in which the patient can make some purposeful reaction to some stimuli. Stupor is a state of motor inactivity and is a feature of catatonia.
B. T.
C. F – Cataplexy is a sudden loss of all movement and muscle tone without associated loss of consciousness and is often associated with narcolepsy. Catalepsy, a synonym for flexibilitas cerea, is a feature of catatonia.
D. T – *Mitgehen* is moving a limb in response to slight pressure on it, despite being told to resist pressure.
E. F – Patients are usually mute, though some may talk nonsense. Verbigeration and *vorbeireden* can occur.

Further reading: Fish (1984; pp. 140–141); Gelder *et al.* (1989; p. 273)

3.22

A. F – Commoner in women.
B. T.
C. T.
D. T.
E. F – Neither the size of the daily dose nor the duration of treatment is associated with the onset of tardive dyskinesia.

Further reading: Gelder *et al.* (1989; pp. 647–649)

3.23 Bleuler's fundamental symptoms of schizophrenia include:
A. Thought disorder.
B. Incongruity of affect.
C. Delusions.
D. Autism.
E. Catatonia.

3.24 The following features are more characteristic of schizophrenia than of mania:
A. Normal syntactic structure.
B. Poverty of speech.
C. Distractible speech.
D. Tangentiality.
E. Pressure of speech.

3.25 Factors associated with a good outcome in schizophrenia include:
A. Previous psychiatric history.
B. Being married.
C. Prominent affective symptoms.
D. Younger age of onset.
E. Insidious onset.

3.23

A. T – The Swiss psychiatrist Eugen Bleuler coined the term schizophrenia in 1911. He distinguished between fundamental and accessory symptoms. Fundamental symptoms included thought disorder, blunting and incongruity of affect, autism and ambivalence. Accessory symptoms included hallucinations, delusions and catatonic phenomena.
B. T.
C. F.
D. T.
E. F.

Further reading: Kendall (1993; pp. 397–398)

3.24

A. F – Syntactic structure in thought-disordered schizophrenics has been shown to be different from normal controls and from manics.
B. T – Poverty of speech and poverty of content of speech occur more frequently in schizophrenics than in manics and normal controls.
C. F – Pressure of speech, clanging, distractible speech or circumstantiality occur more commonly in manics than in thought-disordered schizophrenics.
D. F – Tangentiality has been shown to occur almost equally in schizophrenics and manics.
E. F.

Further reading: Andreasen (1979a, 1979b); Morice and Ingram (1982); Kendall (1993; p. 404)

3.25

A. F – Good outcome is associated with no previous psychiatric history.
B. T.
C. T.
D. F – Older age at onset is associated with good outcome.
E. F – Sudden onset and short duration of episode are associated with a good outcome.

Further reading: Gelder *et al.* (1989; p. 311)

3.26 The following are features of pathological grief and are not seen in normal grief reactions:

A. Feelings of self-reproach.
B. Prolonged/self-punitive grief.
C. Poor memory.
D. Poor concentration.
E. Intense feelings of helplessness.

3.27 The following have been described in mania:

A. Stupor.
B. Schneiderian first-rank symptoms.
C. Delusions of persecution.
D. Nihilistic delusions.
E. Formal thought disorder.

3.28 Secondary mania has been reported in association with the following:

A. Steroids.
B. Levodopa.
C. Bromide.
D. Influenza.
E. Fever.

3.29 Depression:

A. Is a recognized complication of cerebral tumours.
B. Is a common complication of head injury.
C. After a stroke is characteristically associated with lesions of the anterior left hemisphere.
D. After subarachnoid haemorrhage is particularly associated with posterior communicating aneurysms.
E. May occur in neurological disorders with subcortial pathology.

3.26

A. T – Parkes has subdivided pathological grief into three common patterns: the unexpected grief syndrome; the ambivalent grief syndrome and the chronic grief syndrome. Feelings of self reproach are typical of the unexpected grief syndrome.
B. T – Ambivalent grief.
C. F – A feature of normal grief.
D. F – A feature of normal grief.
E. T – A feature of chronic grief.

Further reading: Parkes CM (1985)

3.27

A. T – Rare.
B. T – In 10–20% of manic patients.
C. T – Grandiose and persecutory delusions, also delusions of reference.
D. F – These occur in severe depressive disorder.
E. T – There is flight of ideas, which is a type of formal thought disorder.

Further reading: Gelder *et al.* (1989; pp. 11–12; 223–225)

3.28

A. T.
B. T.
C. T.
D. T.
E. T.

Further reading: Krauthammer and Klerman (1978)

3.29

A. T – Depression and anxiety are common.
B. T – Both neurotic and psychotic depression.
C. F – This case is far from proven. Depression after stroke is probably largely determined by social factors.
D. T – Because rupture interferes with the fine perforating vessels to the hypothalamus.
E. T – For instance, Parkinson's disease.

Further reading: House (1987); Lishman (1987; pp. 165–167, 188, 338); House *et al.* (1991)

3.30 Postnatal depression characteristically:

A. Occurs in about 10–15% of women.
B. Occurs within 6 weeks of childbirth.
C. Is more likely in women who have had an assisted delivery.
D. Is more likely in older women.
E. Is more likely in women from a lower social class.

3.31 Depression in the elderly:

A. May present with somatic complaints.
B. Does not present as a disorder of behaviour.
C. May present as anxiety.
D. Is unrelated to bereavement.
E. Is commonly associated with deficits in higher cortical function.

3.32 Characteristic features of paranoid personality disorder (*DSM-IV*) include:

A. A strong familial association with schizophrenia.
B. Pervasive distrust and suspiciousness of others.
C. A predisposition to jealousy.
D. Persecutory delusions.
E. A reluctance to become close to others.

3.30

A. T – Within 6 weeks of childbirth 10–15% of mothers may become seriously depressed.
B. T – And if untreated can last for 6 months or more.
C. F.
D. F.
E. F.

Further reading: Cox (1993; pp. 578–585)

3.31

A. T – Reported for both inpatient and community samples.
B. F – Food refusal, incontinence, screaming and aggressive behaviour may be the presenting symptoms of elderly people in residential facilities.
C. T – A common accompanying symptom which may dominate the clinical picture.
D. F – Bereavement is a frequent precipitating factor.
E. F – Although 10–20% of depressed elderly patients are found to have a substantial cognitive impairment, deficits in higher cortical function are rarely present.

Further reading: Baldwin (1991; pp. 680–685)

3.32

A. F – There is a familial association but the relationship is weaker than for schizotypal personality disorder.
B. T – These are the central features.
C. T.
D. F – Sometimes their suspicious ideas may be mistaken for persecutory delusions.
E. T.

Further reading: American Psychiatric Association (1994)

3.33 Münchhausen's syndrome
A. Is a term which was coined by Baron von Münchhausen.
B. Is commoner in men.
C. Has a good prognosis.
D. Is classified under malingering in *DSM-IV.*
E. Typically occurs in people who are addicted to opiates.

3.34 Somatic symptoms of anxiety include:
A. Rotational dizziness.
B. Difficulty swallowing.
C. Difficulty exhaling.
D. Blurred vision.
E. Loss of libido.

3.35 The following symptoms are more common in agoraphobia than in other kinds of phobic disorder:
A. Panic attacks.
B. Anticipatory anxiety.
C. Depression.
D. Depersonalization.
E. Obsessional thoughts.

3.33

A. F – It was coined by Asher in 1951, to describe a group of patients who present dramatically to hospitals with histories typical of acute organic emergencies.
B. T.
C. F – The prognosis is uncertain but is likely to be poor. There is no established treatment.
D. F – It is classified under factitious disorder.
E. F – Although pethidine and morphine are commonly demanded for pain relief, dependence on such drugs seems rare.

Further reading: Gelder *et al.* (1989; pp. 418–419)

3.34

A. F – Dizziness is a feature of anxiety but it is not rotational.
B. T – Dry mouth, epigastric discomfort, difficulty swallowing, palpitations, frequency and urgency of micturition are common symptoms.
C. F – Difficulty inhaling is typical. Expiratory difficulty occurs in asthmatics. Hyperventilation is also a feature.
D. T – Blurred vision and tinnitus are also described.
E. F – This is more likely to be a symptom of depression.

Further reading: Gelder *et al.* (1989; pp. 175–178)

3.35

A. T – Anxious cognitions are also common.
B. F – This is a characteristic feature of all phobic disorders.
C. T – Depressive symptoms are common.
D. T – Depersonalization symptoms are also common.
E. T.

Further reading: Gelder *et al.* (1989; pp. 186–188)

3.36 In obsessive-compulsive disorder the obsessional thoughts experienced:
- A. Are usually unpleasant.
- B. Are resisted by the patient.
- C. Intrude forcibly into the mind.
- D. Are recognized by the patient as his or her own thoughts.
- E. May take the form of rhymes.

3.37 The following factors are significantly more common in patients with pseudoseizures (psychogenic seizures; hysterical seizures) than in epileptic controls:
- A. Family history of psychiatric disorder.
- B. Past history of attempted suicide.
- C. Schizophrenia.
- D. Sexual maladjustment.
- E. Aggressive outbursts.

3.38 The following are true of Briquet's syndrome (somatization disorder):
- A. It was described in 1859 by Briquet, a French physician.
- B. Conversion symptoms are essential to the diagnosis.
- C. Somatic complaints often involve the chest and heart.
- D. It runs in families.
- E. Depression is not a feature.

3.36

A. T – They are usually unpleasant and often abhorrent.
B. T – The patient feels compelled to push them out of his or her mind and resist them.
C. T – They are generally experienced as intrusive, forcing themselves on the patient against his or her will; obsessional thoughts may be evoked by external cues or come out of the blue.
D. T – Although they are experienced as absurd, they are hard to drive away, and impair concentration and cause distress.
E. T – Words, phrases or rhymes.

Further reading: Marks (1987; pp. 431–432); Gelder *et al.* (1989; pp. 196–198); Freeman (1993; pp. 504–510)

3.37

A. T – A past history or family history of psychiatric disorder is commoner in patients with pseudoseizures.
B. T – A past history of attempted suicide and current affective disorder is commoner.
C. F – See above.
D. T.
E. F – Not described.

Further reading: Roy (1979); Lishman (1987; pp. 259–261)

3.38

A. F – Briquet wrote a monograph on hysteria in 1859. The St Louis group described the syndrome of multiple somatization disorder and gave it the eponym Briquet's syndrome. It is also known as St Louis hysteria.
B. F – While conversion symptoms occur, they are not essential to the diagnosis.
C. T – e.g. dyspnoea, palpitations, chest pain. Less frequent symptoms include back and joint pain and menstrual symptoms.
D. T – It occurs in 20% of first-degree female relatives of index cases. There is also an excess of alcoholism and psychopathic personality in male relatives of index cases.
E. F – Depression and anxiety are often present.

Further reading: Gelder *et al.* 1989; pp. 206–207); Freeman (1993; pp. 510–511)

3.39 Serotonin (5-HT):
A. Is found only in the brain.
B. Brain levels are raised by MAOIs.
C. Is produced from tyrosine.
D. Is metabolized to 5-HIAA.
E. Is involved in the promotion of wakefulness.

3.40 The following are pharmacological properties of therapeutic concentrations of lithium:
A. Sedation.
B. Depressant.
C. Euphoriant.
D. Mood-stabilizing.
E. Convulsant.

3.41 Recognized effects of antipsychotic agents include:
A. Increase in plasma prolactin.
B. Increase in growth hormone (GH) levels.
C. Blockage of alpha-adrenergic receptors.
D. Akathisia.
E. Hypertension.

3.39

A. F – 95% of total body 5-HT is in the gastrointestinal system and blood platelets; 5% is in the brain, where highest concentrations are in the hypothalamus and limbic system.
B. T – Following inhibition of MAO, brain concentrations of noradrenaline, 5-HT and dopamine rise.
C. F – 5-HT is produced from tryptophan.
D. T.
E. F – 5-HT has widespread effects on vegetative functions such as appetite, sleep and sexual behaviour.

Further reading: Reveley and Campbell (1984; pp. 70–72); Silverstone and Turner (1988; pp. 14, 21–23, 27, 32–36)

3.40

A. F – Lithium is not a sedative, depressant or euphoriant and this differentiates it from other psychotropic agents.
B. F.
C. F.
D. T – The mechanism of action is unknown, although effects on biological membranes and synaptic neurotransmission are suspected.
E. F.

Further reading: Baldessarini (1990; p. 418)

3.41

A. T – Blockade of the tuberoinfundibular dopaminergic system produces an increase in prolactin.
B. F – Neuroleptics tend to decrease serum GH.
C. T – The effects at alpha-adrenergic receptors may contribute to the sedative and hypotensive actions of the antipsychotics.
D. T – Extrapyramidal side-effects are common with antipsychotics. They include parkinsonian symptoms, dystonia, akathisia and tardive dyskinesia.
E. F – Hypotension can occur, especially when the less potent aliphatic or piperidine phenothiazines are given intramuscularly.

Further reading: Campbell and Reveley (1984; pp. 118–121); Silverstone and Turner (1988; pp. 124–129)

3.42 Recognized side-effects of chlorpromazine include:
A. Cholestatic jaundice.
B. A quinidine-like antiarrhythmic effect on the heart.
C. Hypoglycaemia.
D. Amenorrhoea in women.
E. Weight gain.

3.43 Characteristic side-effects of chronic lithium use include:
A. Nephrogenic diabetes insipidus.
B. Increased levels of circulating polymorphonuclear leukocytes.
C. Weight loss.
D. Oedema.
E. Thirst.

3.44 The following antidepressant drugs are potent blockers of 5-HT uptake:
A. Desipramine.
B. Clomipramine.
C. Nortriptyline.
D. Fluoxetine.
E. Mianserin.

3.42

A. T – This is a recognized hypersensitivity reaction occasionally seen and occurs within a few weeks of starting treatment. It was not uncommon when chlorpromazine was first introduced. If it occurs, chlorpromazine should be stopped immediately.

B. T – Chlorpromazine has a direct negative inotropic action and a quinidine-like effect on the heart. ECG changes include prolongation of the Q-T and P-R intervals, S-T depression and T-wave blunting.

C. F – Chlorpromazine may impair glucose tolerance and insulin release to some extent in 'prediabetic' patients. This is not seen with other neuroleptics.

D. T – Chlorpromazine can reduce urinary concentrations of gonadotrophins as well as those of oestrogen and progesterone. This action may contribute to amenorrhoea, sometimes seen in women on chlorpromazine.

E. T – Weight gain and an increase in appetite are seen with all phenothiazines, perhaps less so with haloperidol.

Further reading: Baldessarini (1990; pp. 392–393)

3.43

A. T – This appears to be due to inhibition of vasopressin-sensitive adenylate cyclase within the kidney with a rise in vasopressin levels. Patients complain of thirst and polyuria.

B. T – A benign sustained increase in polymorphonuclear leukocytes occurs and is reversed within a week of termination of treatment.

C. F – Weight gain is usually seen.

D. T.

E. T.

Further reading: Silverstone and Turner (1988; pp. 172–173)

3.44

A. F – Secondary amines are more potent than tertiary amines in blocking noradrenaline uptake.

B. T – Potent and selective inhibitor of 5-HT uptake.

C. F – Preferential action on noradrenaline pathways.

D. T.

E. F.

Further reading: Baldessarini (1990; p. 408)

3.45 Benzodiazepines:
A. Potentiate the actions of GABA at presynaptic and postsynaptic sites.
B. Enhance the sedative effects of antipsychotic drugs.
C. Can cause excessive weight gain.
D. Withdrawal syndrome closely resembles the opiate withdrawal syndrome.
E. Cross the blood–placental barrier.

3.46 The limbic system is made up of the following structures:
A. Dentate gyrus.
B. Parahippocampal gyrus.
C. Subthalamic nucleus.
D. Stria terminalis.
E. Cingulate gyrus.

3.47 The major sources of afferents to the corpus striatum include:
A. Red nucleus.
B. Cerebral cortex.
C. Substantia nigra.
D. Hypothalamus.
E. Septal nuclei.

3.45

A. T.
B. T.
C. T.
D. F – Benzodiazepine withdrawal has many features in common with alcohol withdrawal and closely resembles barbiturate withdrawal. It is distinct from the opiate withdrawal syndrome.
E. T – Readily cross the blood–placental barrier and depress respiration in the newborn.

Further reading: Lader (1987)

3.46

A. T – The dentate gyrus is part of the hippocampal formation.
B. T – The following structures tend to be included in the limbic system: grey matter – limbic lobe (parahippocampal and cingulate gyri), hippocampal formation, part of the amygdaloid nucleus, the hypothalamus (especially mamillary bodies) and anterior nucleus of thalamus; and fibre bundles – fornix, mamillothalamic tract and stria terminalis.
C. F.
D. T.
E. T.

Further reading: Brodal (1981; pp. 689–690); Barr and Kiernan (1988; pp. 266–274)

3.47

A. F.
B. T - The cerebral cortex is the major source of afferents to the striatum (corticostriatal projections).
C. T – The subatantia nigra and thalamus also send important projections (nigrostriatal and thalamostriatal) to the corpus striatum. The fourth important source of afferents is the raphe nuclei.
D. F.
E. F.

Further reading: Brodal (1981; pp. 215–219)

3.48 Characteristic features of the lateral medullary or Wallenberg's syndrome include:

A. Ipsilateral loss of pain and temperature sensibility in the area of distribution of the trigeminal nerve.
B. Contralateral loss of pain and temperature sensibility.
C. Contralateral hemiparesis.
D. Paralysis of tongue muscles.
E. Paralysis of muscles of soft palate on side of lesion.

3.49 Neuropathological features of herpes simplex encephalitis include:

A. Perivascular inflammation with lymphocytes and histiocytes.
B. Subcortical areas are mainly affected.
C. Presence of Cowdry type A inclusion bodies.
D. The parietal region is especially involved.
E. Symmetrical lesions.

3.50 Characteristic pathological features of general paresis include:

A. Neuronal loss.
B. Presence of spirochaetes in brain.
C. Periarteritis and endarteritis of cerebral vessels.
D. Presence of rod cells.
E. Normal-sized brain.

3.48

A. T – Due to involvement of the spinal trigeminal tract and its nucleus.
B. T – Also true, due to interruption of the lateral spinothalamic tract in the spinal lemniscus.
C. F – This is a feature of the medial medullary syndrome.
D. F – Hypoglossal nucleus is not affected.
E. T – Destruction of the nucleus ambiguus causes paralysis of muscles of the soft palate, pharynx and larynx on the side of the lesion, with difficulty in swallowing and phonation.

Further reading: Barr and Kiernan (1988; pp. 117–119)

3.49

A. T – These are non-specific changes characteristic of encephalitis.
B. F – The cerebral cortex is mainly affected in adults.
C. T – These are often detected in the neurones, astrocytes and oligodendrocytes and are large eosinophilic intranuclear masses surrounded by a clear halo and displacing the nucleus to the periphery.
D. F – Medial temporal and orbital regions especially are affected.
E. F – Usually asymmetrical.

Further reading: Lishman (1987; p. 299); Esiri and Kennedy (1992; pp. 346–352)

3.50

A. T – Particularly in the frontal and parietal regions.
B. T – This is the only syphilitic disease in which spirochaetes can be demonstrated in the brain.
C. F – This is a feature of meningovascular syphilis.
D. T – Enlarged microglial cells arranged in rows which stain with Prussian blue because they are impregnated with iron.
E. F – The brain is atrophied.

Further reading: Lishman (1987; pp. 280–281); Reid and Fallon (1992; p. 330)

Paper 4

4.1 The following statements about auditory hallucinations in schizophrenia are correct:

A. The voices are usually in the second or third person.
B. The voices are well-localized in space.
C. The voices increase if sensory input is restricted.
D. Over 90% of schizophrenics will hear voices at some time in their illness.
E. The voices usually decrease if the patient becomes drowsy.

4.2 Haptic hallucinations are:

A. Tactile hallucinations.
B. Autoscopic hallucinations.
C. Typically reflex hallucinations.
D. Sensory hallucinations.
E. Pathognomonic of schizophrenia.

4.3 The following statements are correct:

A. A patient with visual agnosia has adequate eyesight, cannot recognize familiar objects visually, but can recognize them easily when allowed to touch them.
B. Achromatopsia is the same as colour blindness.
C. Auditory agnosia is a form of deafness.
D. In hemisomatagnosia the patient tends to neglect the affected (usually the left) side of the body.
E. Finger agnosia is a form of stereoagnosia.

4.1

A. T.
B. F – The voices are usually poorly localized in space and, even if they are localized, there is no consistent lateralization.
C. T – The voices tend to increase if sensory input is restricted or if the patient is angry, aroused or tense.
D. F – Just over half of patients with schizophrenia will hear voices at some time in their lives.
E. F – The voices usually decrease if the patient listens to meaningful and interesting speech, and, paradoxically increase on becoming drowsy.

Further reading: Cutting (1989)

4.2

A. T – Tactile hallucinations are sometimes called haptic hallucinations.
B. F – This is the experience of seeing one's own body projected into external space.
C. F – This is when a stimulus in one sensory modality results in a hallucination in another. It may occur after taking drugs such as LSD, or rarely in schizophrenia.
D. T.
E. F.

Further reading: Schneider (1959; p. 97); Gelder *et al.* (1989; pp. 8–10)

4.3

A. T.
B. F – Achromatopsia is an acquired colour agnosia. Affected individuals can match objects of the same colour correctly, thus they retain colour vision. They have, however, a visual agnosia affecting the ability to distinguish colours.
C. F – Hearing is normal but the patient cannot recognize familiar sounds such as the jingling of coins.
D. T – This occurs most commonly in patients with threatened or actual *left-sided* hemiplegia; the patient neglects the affected side of the body.
E. F – A form of autotopagnosia confined to the fingers, and a feature of Gerstmann's syndrome.

Further reading: Kräupl-Taylor (1983; pp. 62–64)

4.4 Psychotic delusions are:
A. False convictions.
B. Ego-involved.
C. Idiosyncratic.
D. Incorrigible.
E. Preoccupying.

4.5 The following may occur in delirium:
A. Illusions.
B. Visual hallucinations.
C. Tactile hallucinations.
D. Auditory hallucinations.
E. Persecutory delusions.

4.6 Characteristic features of an epileptic twilight state include:
A. Impaired consciousness.
B. Duration of between 5 minutes and 1 hour.
C. Visual hallucinations.
D. Panic.
E. Psychomotor agitation.

4.4

A. T – Not just false beliefs.
B. T – Infused with a sense of great personal importance.
C. T – Unshared false convictions.
D. T.
E. T – 'The psychotic delusion is an absolute conviction of the truth of a proposition which is idiosyncratic, ego-involved, incorrigible and often preoccupying.'

Further reading: Kräupl-Taylor (1979; pp. 125–130)

4.5

A. T.
B. T – Frequent and may have a fantastic content.
C. T.
D. T.
E. T – Ideas of reference and often persecutory delusions are common, but are usually transient and poorly elaborated.

Further reading: Lishman (1987; p. 5); Gelder *et al.* (1989; pp. 348–349)

4.6

A. T – Consciousness is always impaired.
B. F – Lasts for 1 to several hours and may be prolonged for up to a week or more.
C. T – Usually visual hallucinations are very vivid and highly coloured. Extensive delusions of a paranoid flavour are also common.
D. T – Abnormal affective states occur, which include panic, terror, anger or ecstasy.
E. F – Psychomotor retardation is marked, with marked perseveration of speech.

Further reading: Lishman (1987; pp. 224–225)

4.7 Dysmorphophobia:

A. Is a phobic symptom in phenomenological terms.
B. Usually takes the form of an overvalued idea.
C. May take a delusional form.
D. Can coexist with other psychiatric disorders in the same individual.
E. Can present to plastic surgery clinics.

4.8 Clinical features of the amnesic (Wernicke–Korsakoff) syndrome include:

A. Impairment of recent memory.
B. Aphasia.
C. Peripheral neuropathy.
D. Confabulation in all cases.
E. Ataxia.

4.9 In Freud's theory of development:

A. The oral phase occurs between the ages of 1 and 2.
B. The latency period follows the phallic–Oedipal phase.
C. The anal phase is associated with anxiety about sexual differences.
D. The phallic–Oedipal phase occurs between the ages of 2 and 3.
E. Latency is a period when the gender role is established.

4.7

A. F – Dysmorphophobia is phenomenologically nearer to an obsession or an overvalued idea. Dysmorphophobics are convinced that some part of their body is too large, too small or misshapen. They commonly complain about the nose, but also about the chin, penis, breasts and wrinkles. To others their appearance is within normal limits.
B. T – In patients with a personality disorder the preoccupation is usually an overvalued idea; in those with a psychiatric disorder it is usually delusional.
C. T.
D. T – Typically personality disorder and psychosis.
E. T – Less severe forms tend to present to ear, nose and throat, plastic surgery and dermatology clinics. The more severe cases, described in the psychiatric literature, are rare.

Further reading: Hay (1970); McKenna (1984); Gelder *et al.* (1989; pp. 417–418)

4.8

A. T – An inability to learn new facts.
B. F – The patient is able to hold a conversation.
C. T.
D. F – May be present but is not an essential feature.
E. T – Usually include cerebellar ataxia.

Further reading: Lishman (1987; pp. 491–499); Gelder *et al.* (1989; pp. 354–356)

4.9

A. F – The oral phase occurs between birth and 1 year.
B. T.
C. F – In the anal phase (1–3 years) the infant gets gratification from gaining control over withholding or eliminating faeces. Anxiety about sexual differences occurs in the phallic–Oedipal phase.
D. F – The phallic–Oedipal phase occurs between the ages of 3 and 5 and during this time the child becomes aware of his or her genitalia.
E. F – Latency is a period of relative quiescence of sexual interest which occurs between the phallic–Oedipal phase and puberty.

Further reading: Brown and Pedder (1991; pp. 40–41)

4.10 The following terms are associated with Carl Rogers:
- A. Extraversion.
- B. Accurate empathy.
- C. Individuation.
- D. Genuineness.
- E. Transitional phenomena.

4.11 Defence mechanisms include:
- A. Reaction formation.
- B. Altruism.
- C. Sublimation.
- D. Reconstruction.
- E. Rationalization.

4.12 Curative factors specific for groups include:
- A. Ambition.
- B. Universality.
- C. Altruism.
- D. Release.
- E. Development of socializing techniques.

4.10

A. F – Extraversion was coined by Jung.
B. T – Rogers and his colleagues have shown that effective therapists have three characteristics: accurate empathy, non-possessive warmth and genuineness.
C. F – Jung.
D. T.
E. F – Winnicott described transitional objects and transitional phenomena.

Further reading: Brown and Pedder (1991; pp. 95, 102–103, 107)

4.11

A. T – This is when an unacceptable impulse is mastered by an exaggeration of the opposing tendency, e.g. solicitude as a reaction formation to cruelty.
B. F – This is caring for and helping others in need and is considered by Yalom to be a therapeutic factor in group therapy.
C. T – This was described by Anna Freud as 'the displacement of the instinctual aim in conformity with higher social values'. It is the most advanced and mature defence mechanism and is associated with creativity.
D. F.
E. T – When the subject justifies an unconscious impulse and is unaware of its source.

Further reading: Brown and Pedder (1991; pp. 24–31, 133)

4.12

A. F.
B. T – Yalom described 11 primary curative factors specific to groups. These are installation of hope, universality, imparting of information, interpersonal learning, altruism, the corrective recapitulation of the primary family group, development of socializing techniques, imitative behaviour, group cohesiveness, catharsis and existential factors.
C. T.
D. F.
E. T.

Further reading: Yalom (1985; pp. 3–6)

4.13 In psychoanalytic treatment, the negative therapeutic reaction:

A. Describes the situation in which the patient's condition gets worse, following an awareness by the patient or expression by the therapist of improvement.
B. May occur in patients who have strong guilt feelings.
C. Characteristically occurs at the termination of treatment.
D. Is considered to be a function of the psychoanalytic treatment process.
E. Has been applied extensively outside clinical psychoanalysis.

4.14 Day-dreams

A. Are less easily understood than dreams.
B. Are of no interest in the psychotherapeutic setting.
C. May be escapist fantasies.
D. May be rehearsals for future actions.
E. Are of no importance in cases of people with sexual difficulties.

4.15 Characteristic features of head injuries due to boxing include:

A. Cerebral atrophy on CT scan, showing a significant association with the number of knock-outs sustained.
B. Epilepsy.
C. Cerebellar disorder.
D. Pyramidal disorder.
E. Extrapyramidal disorder.

4.13

A. T – When the patient would normally be expected to experience relief.
B. T – Guilt feelings are evoked by improvement. The patient seeks to reduce these feelings by getting or feeling worse.
C. F – The reasons for a patient relapsing at the time of termination are distinct from the negative therapeutic reaction.
D. F – The propensity for negative therapeutic reactions is considered to be a function of the character of the patient.
E. F – Unlike transference and acting out.

Further reading: Sandler *et al.* (1970g)

4.14

A. F – Although day-dreams are largely emotionally determined, consciousness imposes a certain coherence on them which is lacking in night dreams.
B. F – Everyone day-dreams. In the treatment setting day-dreams can help to shed light upon character.
C. T.
D. T – Or attempts at finding solutions to problems.
E. F – The exploration of day-dreams is especially important in such people.

Further reading: Storr (1979; pp. 49–51)

4.15

A. F – Cerebral atrophy antedating overt signs of brain damage has been shown on CT scan. It is significantly associated with the *number* of bouts fought, not the number of knock-outs. This implies a cumulative effect of multiple subconcussive blows to the head.
B. F – Epilepsy occurred no more frequently in Robert's (1969) series than in the general population.
C. T.
D. T.
E. T.

Further reading: Roberts (1969); Lishman (1987; pp. 173–176)

4.16 Characteristic clinical features of normal pressure hydrocephalus include:

A. Memory impairment.
B. Cerebellar ataxia.
C. Headache.
D. Papilloedema.
E. Normal EEG.

4.17 The following can cause acute organic but not chronic organic reactions:

A. Myxoedema.
B. Hypoglycaemia.
C. Folic acid deficiency.
D. Congestive cardiac failure.
E. Uraemia.

4.18 The following statements concerning hyperparathyroidism are true:

A. Depression is common.
B. The level of psychiatric disturbance is directly related to circulating parathormone levels.
C. The majority of patients first present with psychiatric features.
D. Skull X-ray consistently shows calcification in the basal ganglia.
E. Physical symptoms include increased thirst and polyuria.

4.16

A. T – The characteristic triad includes a slowly progressive gait disorder, urinary incontinence and impairment of mental function. Mental changes usually appear first.
B. F – Frank ataxia is rare. The gait disturbance usually takes the form of unsteadiness and impairment of balance. Other features are difficulty turning and initiating movements.
C. F – Headache is rare and, if present, is usually minimal.
D. F – Does not occur.
E. F – EEG is frequently abnormal, showing non-specific random theta or delta activity.

Further reading: Lishman (1987; pp. 639–644)

4.17

A. F.
B. F.
C. F.
D. F.
E. F.

Note: All of the above can cause acute or chronic organic reactions.

Further reading: Lishman (1987 ; pp. 129–131)

4.18

A. T – Depression and anergia are the commonest psychiatric features. Cognitive impairment also occurs.
B. F – But is related to circulating levels of calcium.
C. F – In the majority of patients physical complaints are the predominant feature. A few present first with psychiatric features, but many realize in retrospect that they have experienced anergia and low spirits for years.
D. F – Skull X-ray may occasionally show calcification in the caudate nuclei and frontal lobes, although this is much less than in hypoparathyroidism, as the calcium deposits are finely distributed.
E. T – Also pain, fracture or deformity of bones, renal colic, muscle weakness, diffuse headache, anorexia and nausea.

Further reading: Lishman (1987; pp. 447–450)

4.19 The following features are characteristic of acute intermittent porphyria:

A. It is inherited as an autosomal recessive gene.
B. It may resemble hysteria.
C. It may be precipitated by carbamazepine.
D. Epileptic seizures occur in some 20% of patients.
E. Psychiatric symptoms may resemble schizophrenia.

4.20 Loosening of associations:

A. Is typical of mania.
B. Includes Knight's move.
C. Occurs in flight of ideas.
D. Was described by Bleuler.
E. Results in perseveration.

4.21 Schneider's first-rank symptoms:

A. Lead to high reliability in the diagnosis of schizophrenia.
B. Are a good predictor of outcome in schizophrenia.
C. Are specific to schizophrenia.
D. Give a narrow definition of schizophrenia.
E. Include third person hallucinations.

4.19

A. F – It is inherited as an autosomal dominant gene with incomplete penetrance.
B. T – The differential diagnosis also includes acute organic reaction or functional psychosis.
C. T – Also acute infection, anaesthesia and certain drugs, including barbiturates, amitriptyline, phenytoin, nitrazepam, steroids, the contraceptive pill, oestrogens, tetracyclines, sulphonamides, dichloralphenazone and methyldopa.
D. T.
E. T.

Further reading: Lishman (1987; pp. 482–485)

4.20

A. F – Occurs most often in schizophrenia.
B. T – This is the transition from one topic to another with no logical relationship between the two.
C. F – In flight of ideas, the patient's thoughts move quickly from one topic to another but the links between the topics can be understood and followed. In loosening of associations there is loss of the normal structure of thinking and the patient appears to be thinking in a muddled fashion.
D. T.
E. F – This is persistent and inappropriate repetition of the same thoughts and occurs in dementia, though is not confined to it.

Further reading: Gelder *et al.* (1989; pp. 10–13)

4.21

A. T.
B. F.
C. F – Can occur in mania.
D. T.
E. T – Of first-rank symptoms, third person hallucinations seem to be least discriminating.

Further reading: Brockington (1986); Gelder *et al.* (1989; pp. 279–281)

4.22 Neuroleptic-treated populations more susceptible to tardive dyskinesia include:

A. Affective illness.
B. Learning disability.
C. The elderly.
D. Men.
E. Caucasians.

4.23 Schneider's first-rank symptoms include:

A. Thought withdrawal.
B. Thought broadcasting.
C. Perplexity.
D. Simple auditory hallucinations.
E. Delusional perception.

4.24 Features of schizophrenic speech in thought-disordered patients include:

A. Abnormal syntactic structure.
B. Reduced quantity of speech.
C. Use of a restricted range of words.
D. The same type/token ratio as normals.
E. A tendency to repetition.

4.22

A. T – Patients with affective illness and mental retardation seem to have a greater susceptibility to tardive dyskinesia than patients with schizophrenia.
B. T.
C. T.
D. F.
E. F – There is no racial selection.

Further reading: Tamminga and Thaker (1989)

4.23

A. T – Thought insertion and thought withdrawal are both considered to be first-rank symptoms.
B. T.
C. F – Perplexity is a second-rank symptom.
D. F – First-rank auditory hallucinations are of three kinds: the voices repeating the patient's thoughts aloud as or after he or she thinks them, or anticipating thoughts; two or more voices discussing the patient or arguing about him or her in the third person; and voices commenting on the subject's thoughts or behaviour, often as a running commentary.
E. T.

Further reading: Schneider (1959; pp. 96, 133–135); Mellor (1970, 1982); Kendall (1993; p. 399)

4.24

A. T.
B. T.
C. T.
D. F – Schizophrenics show a lower type/token ratio (i.e. the ratio between the number of different word types and the total number of words).
E. T – Schizophrenics show a tendency to repeat syllables, words and phrases.

Further reading: Morice and Ingram (1982); Kendall (1993; pp. 404–405)

4.25 The following are associated with late paraphrenia:
A. Female sex.
B. Social deafness.
C. Premorbid paranoid personality disorder.
D. Higher social class.
E. Living in residential accommodation.

4.26 The following are characteristic features of a normal grief reaction :
A. Social withdrawal.
B. Loss of sense of purpose or meaning in life.
C. Persistent sense of the presence of the dead person.
D. Helplessness.
E. Impairment of memory.

4.27 The following statements about bipolar and unipolar affective disorders are true:
A. Relatives of bipolar probands have high rates of both bipolar and unipolar illness.
B. Bipolar disorder is more genetic than unipolar disorder.
C. Relatives of unipolar probands have high rates of both bipolar and unipolar illness.
D. Relatives of bipolar probands have a higher rate of affective illness than relatives of unipolar probands.
E. The morbid risk in the general population for severe unipolar disorder is in the range of 3%.

4.25

A. T – Possible protective role of oestrogens, lost after the menopause, together with speculated relative excess of D_2 receptors.
B. T – Conductive hearing loss, contracted in early life, of a degree that impedes social interaction (social deafness) is a risk factor.
C. T – Paranoid and/or schizoid premorbid personalities are commonly found in patients with paraphrenia.
D. F.
E. F.

Further reading: Naguib and Levy (1991; pp. 766–769)

4.26

A. T.
B. T – Also impairment in concentration and memory, lasting feelings of dejection and often disturbances in appetite, weight and sleep.
C. F – A feature of the unexpected grief syndrome which makes it hard for the bereaved person to come to terms with his or her loss.
D. F – Intense feelings of helplessness are associated with chronic grief.
E. T.

Further reading: Parkes CM (1985)

4.27

A. T.
B. T – There is a strong genetic component to affective illness overall. Reanalysis of previous twin studies in terms of the unipolar/bipolar dichotomy suggests that bipolar disorder is more genetic.
C. F – Relatives of unipolar probands have a high risk of unipolar disorder only.
D. T.
E. T – And the morbid risk in the general population for bipolar disorder is less than 1%.

Further reading: Bertelsen *et al.* (1977); Murray and McGuffin (1993; pp. 240–243)

4.28 The following are true of secondary mania:
A. The average age of onset is later than in primary mania.
B. Family history of affective disorder is present in over 85% of cases.
C. There is typically a negative premorbid history.
D. It has been described postoperatively.
E. It has been described in association with treatment with steroids.

4.29 The following are true of seasonal affective disorder:
A. It does not exist in bipolar form.
B. It may exist in a subsyndromal form.
C. Full summer remission occurs in most patients.
D. Bright light treatment is as effective as summer light.
E. Bright light treatment reduces total sleep time.

4.30 Recognized factors associated with persistent mood abnormalities in patients with affective disorder include:
A. Female sex.
B. Greater prevalence of previous thyroid dysfunction.
C. Length of time between onset of depressive symptoms and introduction of treatment.
D. Alcohol abuse.
E. Inadequate treatment.

4.28

A. T – In secondary mania the average age of onset is later than in primary mania.
B. F – This is true for primary mania.
C. T.
D. T.
E. T.

Further reading: Krauthammer and Klerman (1978)

4.29

A. F – Both bipolar (summer mania or hypomania) and unipolar forms exist.
B. T – In the subsyndromal form, winter vegetative symptoms occur without the additional symptoms needed to meet criteria for a diagnosis of major depression.
C. T – When followed prospectively, most subjects remit. Remission is associated with improvement in personality and biological measures.
D. F – Summer light is up to 10 times stronger than currently available light boxes. Lights are not as effective as summer light itself.
E. T – Bright light treatment also increases delta sleep.

Further reading: Lahmeyer and Lilie (1991)

4.30

A. T – Patients with chronic primary major depression are more likely to be female.
B. T.
C. T – Currently the most powerful predictor of chronicity.
D. T – This is a secondary complication, arising after the onset of the depression. Other secondary complications include family or social difficulties, physical illness and drug abuse.
E. T – Inappropriate and inadequate treatment and non-compliance with treatment have also been described.

Further reading: Scott (1988); Scott *et al.* (1991)

4.31 Suicide rates:

A. Are highest in the months of April, May and June in the southern hemisphere.
B. Are lowest in social class V.
C. Are lowest amongst the married.
D. For young men aged 15 to 44 in England and Wales rose by a third between 1980 and 1990.
E. Are highest in elderly men overall in England and Wales.

4.32 DSM-IV Cluster B Personality Disorders include:

A. Histrionic personality disorder.
B. Passive-aggressive personality disorder.
C. Borderline personality disorder.
D. Narcissistic personality disorder.
E. Paranoid personality disorder.

4.31

A. F – Suicide rates show a seasonal variation, with rates being highest in the *spring and early summer* in both northern and southern hemispheres.
B. F – Rates are higher in social classes I and V than in the remaining social classes.
C. T – And increase progressively through the never married, widowed and divorced.
D. T – Most of this change was due to an increase of 78% in those aged 14 to 24.
E. T – The overall rate of suicide remains highest in men aged 75 and over, although in terms of absolute numbers more deaths occur in the younger age groups.

Further reading: Gelder *et al.* (1989; pp. 479–491); Hawton (1992); Gunnell and Frankel (1994)

4.32

A. T – In *DSM-IV* the Personality Disorders are grouped into three clusters based on descriptive similarities. Cluster A includes the Paranoid, Schizoid and Schizotypal Personality Disorders. Cluster B includes the Antisocial, Borderline, Histrionic and Narcissistic Personality Disorders. Cluster C includes the Avoidant, Dependent and Obsessive-Compulsive Personality Disorders.
B. F.
C. T.
D. T.
E. F.

Further reading: American Psychiatric Association (1994)

4.33 Characteristic features of anorexia nervosa include:

A. Amenorrhoea in females.
B. Loss of appetite.
C. Distortion of body image.
D. Recurrent episodes of binge eating.
E. Alcohol abuse.

4.34 Characteristic features of sleep disturbance in generalized anxiety disorder include:

A. Initial insomnia.
B. Night terrors.
C. Waking unrefreshed.
D. Early morning wakening.
E. Unpleasant dreams.

4.33

A. T – This is an important feature which occurs early in the development of the condition and reflects a widespread endocrine disorder involving the hypothalamic–pituitary–gonadal axis. For a definite diagnosis the following are also required (*ICD-10*): body weight is maintained 15% below that expected; weight loss is induced by avoidance of fattening foods and one or more of the following: self-induced vomiting, self-induced purging, excessive exercise, use of appetite suppressants and/or diuretics; body image distortion; and delay in the sequence of pubertal events, if the onset is prepubertal.
B. F – They limit their daily calorie intake because of their intense fear of becoming overweight.
C. T.
D. F – Up to 50% of individuals with anorexia nervosa have episodes of binge eating, but this is not one of the diagnostic criteria. It is a central feature of bulimia nervosa.
E. F.

Further reading: Treasure (1992); World Health Organization (1992)

4.34

A. T – Typically the patient lies awake worrying.
B. T – The patient may wake up during a nightmare or night terrors.
C. T – Patients also wake intermittently throughout the night.
D. F – Should suggest the possibility that anxiety symptoms are secondary to depressive disorder.
E. F.

Further reading: Gelder *et al.* (1989; pp. 176–178)

4.35 The following apply to agoraphobia:
A. It typically begins in the early teenage years.
B. It is commoner in men than in women.
C. Symptoms are reported to diminish with MAOI drugs.
D. The course may be chronic.
E. The treatment of choice is aversion therapy.

4.36 The following features have been described in obsessive-compulsive disorder:
A. Anxiety.
B. Depression.
C. Depersonalization.
D. Grandiose delusions.
E. Autistic thinking.

4.37 Characteristic features of psychogenic blindness include:
A. Abnormal pupillary reflexes.
B. Abnormal visual evoked responses.
C. Tunnel vision.
D. Visual hallucinations.
E. Usually worse at night.

4.35

A. F – Most cases begin in the early or mid 20s, though there is a further period of high onset in the mid 30s.
B. F – Prevalence amongst women is about twice that in men.
C. T.
D. T.
E. F – The treatment of choice is behaviour therapy, combining exposure to phobic situations with training in coping with panic attacks.

Further reading: Gelder *et al.* (1989; pp. 186–190)

4.36

A. T – A prominent symptom.
B. T – Depression is the most common complication, but suicide is rare.
C. T – A proportion of patients with obsessive-compulsive disorder report depersonalization.
D. F – These are a feature of hypomania.
E. F – This is one of Bleuler's fundamental symptoms of schizophrenia.

Further reading: Marks (1987; p. 445); Gelder *et al.* (1989; pp. 196–202); Freeman (1993; pp. 504–510)

4.37

A. F – The pupillary reflexes are preserved.
B. F – These are usually normal.
C. T – While tunnel vision is the commonest pattern of field effect, other patterns can also occur and findings on perimetry are variable.
D. F – Visual hallucinations may indicate a psychotic state, of schizophrenic, affective or organic origin. In non-psychotic individuals with visual hallucinations, physical illness and toxic effects of drugs (tricyclic antidepressants, bromocriptine, anticholinergic agents) should be suspected.
E. F – This is not described.

Further reading: Morgan (1983; pp. 35–36); Gelder *et al.* (1989; pp. 205–206)

4.38 The following are inhibitory amino acids:
A. Glutamic acid.
B. Glycine.
C. Aspartic acid.
D. Adenosine.
E. Tyrosine.

4.39 Recognized side-effects of clozapine include:
A. Neutropenia.
B. Hypersalivation.
C. Urinary incontinence.
D. Myocarditis.
E. Delirium.

4.40 The following antidepressants have sedative properties:
A. Amitriptyline.
B. Imipramine.
C. Trazodone.
D. Fluoxetine.
E. Doxepin.

4.38

A. F – Glutamic acid is an excitatory amino acid and is now established as an excitatory neurotransmitter in the CNS.
B. T – Glycine probably acts as a postsynaptic inhibitory transmitter on motoneurones.
C. F – Aspartic acid is formed from glutamate by transamination with oxalate. It has a central excitatory effect.
D. T.
E. F – However, taurine probably has an inhibitory effect.

Further reading: Reveley and Campbell (1984; p. 74); Silverstone and Turner (1988; pp. 16–17)

4.39

A. T – And a potentially fatal agranulocytosis.
B. T.
C. T.
D. T.
E. T.

Further reading: *British National Formulary* (1994; p. 154)

4.40

A. T.
B. F.
C. T.
D. F – The selective serotonin reuptake inhibitors are less sedative than the tricyclics.
E. T.

Further reading: Baldessarini (1990; p. 407); *British National Formulary* (1994; pp. 162–170)

4.41 Recognized side-effects of chlorpromazine include:
A. Cholestatic jaundice.
B. Prolongation of the P-R and Q-T intervals on the ECG.
C. Hypoglycaemia.
D. Amenorrhoea in women.
E. Weight gain.

4.42 Lithium:
A. Binds to plasma proteins.
B. Is excreted mainly in the urine.
C. Is excreted in breast milk.
D. Is reabsorbed mainly by the distal renal tubules.
E. Does not pass the blood–brain barrier.

4.41

A. T – This is a recognized hypersensitivity reaction occasionally seen and occurs within a few weeks of starting treatment. If it occurs, chlorpromazine should be stopped immediately.

B. T – ECG changes include prolongation of the Q-T and P-R intervals, S-T depression and blunting of T waves.

C. F – Chlorpromazine may impair glucose tolerance and insulin release to some degree in some 'prediabetic' patients. This is not seen with other neuroleptics.

D. T – Chlorpromazine can reduce urinary concentrations of gonadotrophins as well as those of oestrogen and progesterone. This action may contribute to amenorrhoea sometimes seen in women on chlorpromazine.

E. T – Weight gain and an increase in appetite are seen with all phenothiazines.

Further reading: Baldessarini (1990; pp. 392–393)

4.42

A. F – There is no evidence for this.

B. T – Approximately 95% of a single dose of lithium is eliminated in the urine. About one- to two-thirds of an acute oral dose is excreted during a 6–12-hour initial phase of excretion, followed by a slow excretion over the next 10–14 days. Elimination half-life averages 12–24 hours.

C. T.

D. F – 80% of filtered lithium is reabsorbed by the proximal renal tubules. Some reabsorption may occur in the distal tubules.

E. F – However, passage through the blood–brain barrier is slow.

Further reading: Baldessarini (1990; pp. 419–420)

4.43 Recognized effects of benzodiazepines in humans include:
A. Anterograde amnesia.
B. Analgesic action after oral administration.
C. Induction of liver microsomal enzymes.
D. Anticonvulsant activity.
E. No effect on psychomotor function.

4.44 Fenfluramine:
A. Is chemically similar to amphetamine.
B. Has sedative properties.
C. Acts primarily on the dopamine pathways.
D. Has anorectic activity which resides in the L-isomer.
E. Increases uptake of glucose into muscle cells.

4.45 Treatment with lithium carbonate should be avoided or used with caution in the following:
A. Addison's disease.
B. Cardiac disease.
C. Renal impairment.
D. Myasthenia gravis.
E. Pregnancy.

4.43

A. T – The main effects are as follows: sedation, hypnosis, muscle relaxation, anterograde amnesia and anticonvulsant activity.
B. F – Transient analgesia is apparent in humans after intravenous administration.
C. F.
D. T.
E. F.

Further reading: Rall (1990; pp. 346–349); Tyrer and Murphy (1987)

4.44

A. T.
B. T.
C. F – Acts mainly on the 5-HT pathway.
D. F – Its total anorectic activity resides in the D-isomer.
E. T – This peripheral action may play a part in its efficacy in treating obesity.

Further reading: Silverstone and Turner (1988; pp. 243–244, 249)

4.45

A. T – Because of sodium imbalance.
B. T.
C. T.
D. T.
E. T – Not advised during pregnancy, especially during the first trimester.

Further reading: Silverstone and Turner (1988; pp. 173–174); ***British National Formulary*** (1994; pp. 161–162)

4.46 The following structures are seen in the pons:

A. Motor nucleus of the trigeminal nerve.
B. Facial motor nucleus.
C. Trapezoid body.
D. Nucleus ambiguus.
E. Inferior olive.

4.47 A complete third cranial nerve palsy results in:

A. Loss of light reflex in the affected eye.
B. Constriction of the pupil in the affected eye.
C. Preservation of the power of accommodation in the affected eye.
D. Ptosis of the lid of the affected eye.
E. Lateral strabismus in the affected eye.

4.46

A. T – The pons lies between the medulla and the midbrain and is about 2.5 cm in length. It contains the spinal trigeminal tract and nucleus, the pontine trigeminal nucleus, the trigeminal motor nucleus, the abducens nucleus and the motor nucleus of the facial nerve.
B. T.
C. T.
D. F – The nucleus ambiguus and inferior olivary nucleus are found in the medulla.
E. F – But the superior olivary nucleus is located in the pons.

Further reading: Barr and Kiernan (1988; pp. 88, 102–108)

4.47

A. T – Direct and consensual reflexes are lost in the affected eye but preserved in the unaffected eye. Accommodation is also lost in the affected eye.
B. F – The pupil of the affected eye is dilated due to: interruption of the parasympathic fibres and unopposed action of the dilator pupillae muscle, which has sympathetic innervation.
C. F.
D. T – There is marked ptosis due to paralysis of the levator palpebrae.
E. T – Due to unopposed action of the lateral rectus muscle.

Further reading: Barr and Kiernan (1988; pp. 122–123)

4.48 Recognized features of the Brown-Séquard syndrome include:

A. Contralateral spastic paralysis below lesion.
B. Contralateral loss of muscle and joint position sense below lesion.
C. Contralateral loss of pain and temperature sensation below lesion.
D. Incontinence of urine.
E. Contralateral loss of light touch below lesion.

4.49 Recognized features of the normal ageing process include:

A. Senile plaques in all layers of the cortex.
B. Neurofibrillary changes.
C. Neuronal degeneration.
D. Granulovacuolar degeneration.
E. Balloon cells.

4.50 Characteristic pathological features of Creutzfeldt–Jakob disease include:

A. Relative sparing of the parietal and occipital lobes.
B. Degeneration of the corpus callosum.
C. Spongiform degeneration of grey matter.
D. Neurofibrillary tangles.
E. Astrocytic proliferation.

4.48

A. F – In the Brown-Séquard syndrome (hemisection of the spinal cord), the spastic paralysis below the level of the lesion is ipsilateral.
B. F – Posterior column damage causes ipsilateral loss of vibration sense, position sense and tactile discrimination below the injury.
C. T – Contralateral pain and temperature sensation loss below the level of the lesion are due to interruption of the spinothalamic tract.
D. F – Functions of the bladder, rectum and genital organs are usually preserved (bilateral innervation).
E. F – Light touch is not much affected because of bilateral conduction.

Further reading: Brodal (1981; p. 252); Barr and Kiernan (1988; pp. 81–82)

4.49

A. F – Senile plaques are only seen in superficial layers in the normal ageing brain.
B. T.
C. T.
D. T.
E. F – Balloon cells are a feature of Pick's disease.

Further reading: Lishman (1987; pp. 375–377); Tomlinson (1992; pp. 1290–1317)

4.50

A. T – The cortex is nearly always involved in this disease, but the parietal and occipital lobes are often relatively spared.
B. F.
C. T – Creutzfeldt–Jakob is one of the spongiform encephalopathies, and is characterized by the histological triad of neuronal degeneration, astrocytic proliferation and spongiform degeneration of the grey matter.
D. F.
E. T.

Further reading: Lishman (1987; pp. 400–404); Tomlinson (1992; pp. 1366–1375)

Paper 5

5.1 In alcoholic hallucinosis the voices heard:

A. Are usually well-localized.
B. Respond well to neuroleptics.
C. Decrease with drowsiness.
D. Have the same quality as voices encountered in schizophrenic patients.
E. Usually echo the patient's own thoughts.

5.2 According to Schneider, delusional perception:

A. Is often preceded by a delusional atmosphere.
B. Occurs when the individual is in an aroused emotional state.
C. Is made up of two stages.
D. May occur as a delusional memory.
E. Occurs in normal people.

5.3 The following are examples of illusions:

A. Mirage.
B. Eidetic images.
C. Diplopia.
D. *Jamais vu*.
E. Macropsia.

5.1

A. T – There is usually only one voice and the speaker is often identified.
B. F – These voices respond poorly to neuroleptics but clear if the patient remains abstinent from alcohol.
C. F – These voices increase with drowsiness and meaningful noise, suggesting that they are false perceptions of environmental sounds.
D. F – See A, B, C, E.
E. F – This is a first-rank symptom of schizophrenia.

Further reading: Cutting (1989)

5.2

A. T – The delusional atmosphere is vague. The mood of the atmosphere is often referred to as delusional mood.
B. F – Is not derived from any particular emotional state.
C. T – First, the object is perceived and, second, the perceived object is invested with some abnormal significance, usually with self-reference.
D. T – A delusional perception of the past can be a kind of delusional memory, e.g. when a meaning is attached subsequently to a remembered perception.
E. F – Schneider considered that it was 'always a schizophrenic symptom', but could also occur with 'epileptic twilight states, toxic psychoses and morbid cerebral changes'.

Further reading: Schneider (1959; pp. 104–116); Sims (1988; pp. 87–90)

5.3

A. T – A normal illusion.
B. F – These are more or less accurate peripheral replicas of objects which have been attentively observed: they are hallucinations.
C. T – A pathological illusion.
D. T – *Déjà vu* is an illusion of familiarity and *jamais vu* is an illusion of unfamiliarity.
E. T – Objects look abnormally large.

Note: Illusions are misperceptions of external stimuli. They can occur in normal people, in delirium and depression. Psychotic delusions may give rise to delusional illusions, but in practice it is difficult to discern these.

Further reading: Kräupl-Taylor (1979; pp. 100–104); Sims (1988; pp. 65–67)

5.4 Characteristic features of frontal lobe syndrome include:
A. Disinhibition.
B. Depression.
C. Impaired insight.
D. Amnesic syndrome.
E. Right–left disorientation.

5.5 The following psychological symptoms can occur as the predominant feature of a partial seizure of temporal lobe origin:
A. Forced thinking.
B. Ecmnesic hallucinations.
C. Visual hallucinations.
D. Depersonalization.
E. Dysphasia.

5.6 The following are more likely to be features of an acute organic psychosis than acute schizophrenia:
A. Misidentification of persons.
B. Visual hallucinations.
C. Auditory hallucinations.
D. Clear consciousness.
E. Absence of delusions.

5.4

A. T – The personality is profoundly affected in frontal lobe syndrome. Typically the patient lacks initiative and spontaneity and shows reduced motor activity. Social awareness and behaviour are markedly impaired, as is judgement.
B. F – Usually mildly euphoric. There is a tendency to joke and engage in pranks (*Witzelsucht*). True depression is rare.
C. T.
D. F – A feature of bilateral medial temporal lobe lesion.
E. F – A feature of a dominant parietal lobe lesion.

Further reading: Lishman (1987; pp. 68–69); Gelder *et al.* (1989; pp. 356–358)

5.5

A. T – The subject may feel compelled to think about particular subjects, such as death.
B. T – Previous experiences are recalled by the subject and relived with great intensity.
C. T – Simple and complex visual and auditory hallucinations occur, also hallucinations of taste and smell.
D. T – Feelings of depersonalization and derealization may be marked.
E. T – Dysphasia as part of an aura indicates a left temporal lobe focus.

Further reading: Lishman (1987; pp. 218–220); Fenton (1993; p. 347)

5.6

A. T – This is more likely to occur in organic psychosis because of the impaired consciousness, thinking, concentration and attention, also distorted visual perception.
B. T – Although visual hallucinations can occur in schizophrenia, they are more frequent in acute organic psychosis.
C. F.
D. F – This is a feature of acute schizophrenia. Impairment of consciousness is an important feature of acute organic psychosis, though occasionally it is difficult to establish.
E. T – Ideas of reference and delusions are common in acute organic psychosis, but they are commoner in acute schizophrenia.

Further reading: Cutting (1987); Gelder *et al.* (1989; pp. 348–350)

5.7 Overvalued ideas:

A. Were first described by Wernicke.
B. Are firmly held false beliefs.
C. Are partial delusions.
D. May be true or false.
E. May be persecutory in nature.

5.8 The following delusions typically occur in psychotic depression:

A. Delusions of guilt.
B. Delusions of reference.
C. Delusions of persecution.
D. Delusions of thought withdrawal.
E. Delusions of influence.

5.9 In the basic model of psychoanalytic technique:

A. The patient will be encouraged to talk as freely as possible.
B. The major therapeutic interventions of the psychoanalyst are interpretations, confrontations and clarifications.
C. The therapist experiences transference.
D. The working relationship has been referred to as acting out.
E. Resistance is typically experienced by the therapist.

5.7

A. T – In 1900.
B. F – An overvalued idea is an isolated preoccupying belief which is neither delusional nor obsessional in nature.
C. F – Partial delusions are sometimes used to describe beliefs which were held to a delusional extent when the patient was ill, but are doubted on recovery.
D. T.
E. T – Difficult to distinguish from delusions.

Further reading: Gelder *et al.* (1989; pp. 14–15); Fish (1984; p. 45); McKenna (1984)

5.8

A. T – Delusions of guilt and deserved punishment.
B. T.
C. T.
D. F.
E. F – D and E occur in schizophrenia.

Further reading: Kräupl-Taylor (1983; pp. 75–78)

5.9

A. T.
B. T.
C. F – The patient experiences transference.
D. F – The working relationship has been referred to as the therapeutic alliance or the working alliance.
E. F – No, by the patient.

Further reading: Sandler *et al.* (1970a)

5.10 The following are correctly paired:

A. Adler: importance of aggressive strivings and the drive to power.
B. Object relations theorists: prominence of a general life force or libido.
C. Bowlby: attachment.
D. Harlow: curiosity and exploratory drive.
E. Freud: infantile sexuality.

5.11 The following terms are associated with Jung:

A. Introversion.
B. Individual psychology.
C. Collective unconsciousness.
D. Projection.
E. The Shadow.

5.12 The following terms are associated with Alfred Adler:

A. Inferiority complex.
B. Ego psychology.
C. Individuation.
D. 'Masculine protest' in women.
E. Gestalt therapy.

5.10

A. T.
B. F – This is associated with Freud and Jung. Object relations theorists have suggested that the primary motivational drive in humans is to seek relationship with others.
C. T – Bowlby considered attachment as an important primary drive in higher primates, including humans.
D. F – In her work on infant chimpanzees, Harlow showed the drive for attachment to objects (holding having primacy over feeding). Piaget has described curiosity and exploratory drive.
E. T.

Further reading: Brown and Pedder (1991; pp. 31–37)

5.11

A. T – Jung derived the concepts of introversion and extraversion.
B. F – Individual psychology is associated with Adler. Jung developed his own school of analytical psychology.
C. T – Jung was concerned with the interpretation of unconscious material as represented in myths, dreams and culture. His theory incorporates three levels of the psyche: the Conscious, the Personal Unconscious and the Collective Unconscious. He described Archetypes (generalized symbols and images within the Collective Unconscious) which include the Animus and Anima, the Shadow, the Great Mother, the Wise Old Man and the Hero.
D. F – This is one of the nine mechanisms of defence described by Anna Freud in 1936.
E. T – Unacknowledged aspects of the self.

Further reading: Brown and Pedder (1991; pp. 102–103)

5.12

A. T.
B. F – Adler is associated with individual psychology and Anna Freud with ego psychology.
C. F – Jung saw treatment as a process of individuation.
D. T – Adler saw this as a reaction to women's inferior position in society.
E. F – Gestalt therapy was developed by Fritz Perls.

Further reading: Brown and Pedder (1991; pp. 102–105)

5.13 The following are similarities between supportive and exploratory psychotherapy:

A. Unburdening of problems.
B. Confrontation of defences.
C. Regression allowed within sessions.
D. Discussion of problems.
E. Support within the working alliance.

5.14 The following are elements of psychoanalytic psychotherapy:

A. The therapist gives active encouragement and advice.
B. Transference phenomena are explored.
C. The patient is encouraged to talk in an unstructured way.
D. Working through.
E. Role-playing.

5.15 After head injury:

A. The risk of suicide is increased.
B. The presence of neurotic symptoms correlates with the extent of brain damage sustained.
C. Personality change can occur in the absence of brain damage.
D. The incidence of schizophrenia-like psychoses is greater than chance expectation.
E. Hypomania is commoner than depressive psychosis.

5.13

A. T – Unburdening of problems, ventilation of feelings and discussion of current problems occur in both supportive and exploratory psychotherapy.
B. F – Confrontation of defences takes place in exploratory psychotherapy. In supportive psychotherapy defences are supported and reinforced.
C. F – Regression is allowed within sessions in exploratory psychotherapy but is discouraged in supportive psychotherapy.
D. T.
E. T.

Further reading: Brown and Pedder (1991; p. 100)

5.14

A. F – The therapist remains neutral.
B. T – Transference phenomena are explored.
C. T – Free association.
D. T – Elaboration of insights into various areas of the patient's functioning.
E. F.

Further reading: Brown and Pedder (1991; pp. 110–118)

5.15

A. T – Suicide accounts for up to 14% of deaths amongst patients with head injury.
B. F.
C. T – These changes include fluctuating depression, morbid anxiety, obsessional traits and persistent irritability, all of which are common.
D. T – The trauma of the head injury is thought to be of direct aetiological significance.
E. F – Depressive psychosis is much more common after head injury than hypomania.

Further reading: Davison and Bagley (1969); Lishman (1987; pp. 160–168)

5.16 Characteristic clinical features of Creutzfeldt–Jakob disease include:

A. Parietal lobe symptoms.
B. Cortical blindness.
C. Poorly developed or complete loss of alpha rhythms on the EEG.
D. Myoclonic jerks.
E. Preservation of speech.

5.17 Characteristic features of Addison's disease include:

A. Depressive psychosis.
B. Apathy.
C. Hypertension.
D. Memory difficulties.
E. Overactivity.

5.18 Characteristic features of hepatic encephalopathy include:

A. Impaired consciousness.
B. Visual hallucinations.
C. Appearance of delta waves on the EEG.
D. Choreoathetoid movements.
E. Fluctuating neurological disturbance.

5.16

A. T – For instance, right–left disorientation, dyscalculia and finger agnosia.
B. T.
C. F – The EEG in Creutzfeldt–Jakob disease shows a characteristic pattern of triphasic sharp wave complexes, superimposed on progressive suppression of cortical background activity.
D. T – Myoclonic jerks are frequently seen and epileptic fits may occur.
E. F – Speech disturbances are common, with dysphasia and dysarthria.

Further reading: Lishman (1987; pp. 400–404)

5.17

A. F – While depression is a common psychiatric symptom, psychotic features are rare, in contrast with Cushing's syndrome.
B. T – Common and characterized by depression, emotional withdrawal, apathy, loss of drive and initiative.
C. F – Hypotension is almost always present.
D. T – Reported in up to three-quarters of cases.
E. F – Tiredness is an almost universal complaint.

Further reading: Lishman (1987; pp. 439–440)

5.18

A. T – Impaired consciousness is always present during episodes of the disorder. It starts often with hypersomnia and daytime sleepiness, progressing to periods of marked confusion, semicoma or coma.
B. T – These are often very frightening.
C. F – Theta waves replace alpha activity as consciousness becomes impaired. Characteristic triphasic waves, indicating a poor prognosis, are seen later.
D. F – Seen in Wilson's disease. The motor abnormalities of hepatic encephalopathy include a mild exaggeration of tendon reflexes, unobtrusive tremor, a blank or grimacing facial expression and characteristic flapping tremor (asterixis).
E. T.

Further reading: Lishman (1987; pp. 480–482)

5.19 Acute organic reactions are characterized by:
A. A degree of impairment of consciousness.
B. Poverty of thought.
C. Perceptual disturbances.
D. Apathy.
E. Disorientation.

5.20 In Cushing's syndrome:
A. Psychiatric disturbance has been reported in over 50% of cases.
B. Paranoid symptoms are the most frequent psychiatric symptoms.
C. Depression has been reported as particularly common in patients with a pituitary origin of disease.
D. Acute organic reactions are common.
E. CT scanning has shown cerebral atrophy.

5.19

A. T – Careful observation will reveal this. Fluctuation in consciousness from time to time is also an important observation. Often nocturnal worsening occurs.

B. F – Patients have rich, intrusive fantasies. Poverty of thought is more characteristic of chronic organic reactions.

C. T – Perceptual disturbances/distortions, including illusions and visual hallucinations.

D. F – Emotional rapport can usually be established, with patients showing clouding of consciousness. Emotional disturbances seen in acute organic reactions include fear, tension, perplexity and agitation.

E. T.

Further reading: Lishman (1987; pp. 127–133)

5.20

A. T.

B. F – Depressive symptoms are the most frequent psychiatric symptoms, although paranoid features are common. Emotional lability and acute anxiety are also seen.

C. T.

D. F – They are rare.

E. T.

Further reading: Lishman (1987; pp. 436–439)

5.21 Feighner criteria:

A. Demand 6 months' continuous illness for a diagnosis of schizophrenia.

B. Describe a broad definition of schizophrenia.

C. Are good at identifying patients with a poor prognosis.

D. Were developed in Iowa.

E. Are determined using the Schizophrenia and Affective Disorders Schedule (SADS).

5.22 The following statements regarding operationalized definitions of schizophrenia are true:

A. *DSM-IV* criteria are restrictive.

B. The CATEGO computer program incorporates a Schneiderian concept of schizophrenia.

C. Schneider's first-rank symptoms are good at predicting long-term prognosis.

D. The St Louis criteria demand that the subject should have been psychotic for 6 months.

E. The RDC definition demands a 6-month duration of symptoms.

5.21

A. T – The subject should have been continuously ill, though not necessarily psychotic, for at least 6 months and should not have prominent manic or depressive symptoms. The only psychotic symptoms required are delusions or hallucinations of almost any type, or clear-cut thought disorder. At least three of five characteristics must also be present for a diagnosis of definite schizophrenia: single; poor premorbid social adjustment; family history of schizophrenia; absence of alcoholism or drug abuse within 1 year of psychosis; and onset of illness under the age of 40.

B. F – No, they are restrictive.

C. T.

D. F – In St Louis. They are sometimes referred to as the St Louis criteria.

E. F – This has been developed for use with Research Diagnostic Criteria (RDC).

Further reading: Feighner *et al.* (1972); Spitzer *et al.* (1978); Endicott and Spitzer (1978)

5.22

A. T – *DSM-IV*, like the St Louis criteria, requires that continuous signs of the disturbance persist for at least 6 months, therefore defining a group of patients with a poor long-term prognosis.

B. T – CATEGO criteria are broader. They are poor at predicting outcome because no account is taken of symptom duration or the presence of affective symptoms.

C. F – Schneiderian first-rank symptoms are reliably rated, but poor at predicting long-term prognosis.

D. F – The St Louis criteria demand that the patient should have been 'continuously ill' for 6 months, although not necessarily psychotic, and should not have prominent manic or depressive symptoms.

E. F – RDC criteria demand a 2-week duration of symptoms but require the presence of thought disorder and hallucinations and delusions of particular kinds.

Further reading: Feighner *et al.* (1972); Wing *et al.* (1974); Endicott and Spitzer (1978); Spitzer *et al.* (1978); American Psychiatric Association (1994); Kendall (1993; pp. 397–426)

5.23 The following statements regarding Capgras syndrome are true:

A. The patient believes that a person familiar to him or her has been replaced by a double with the same, or virtually the same, physical appearance.
B. It is commoner in women than in men.
C. It is a delusional memory.
D. It is commonly associated with schizophrenia.
E. Whenever there is evidence of cerebral dysfunction, it always includes, or is restricted to, the left hemisphere.

5.24 The following are true of schizophrenia:

A. The incidence is fairly stable across a wide range of cultures, climates and ethnic groupings.
B. It is commoner in women.
C. It is associated with summer birth.
D. There is a positive association with rheumatoid arthritis.
E. The incidence is higher in the unmarried than the married.

5.25 Studies of schizophrenia show that:

A. The course and outcome are similar in different countries.
B. There is an increase in life events in the 3 weeks before the onset of acute symptoms in first episodes only.
C. An understimulating hospital environment is associated with the clinical poverty syndrome.
D. Neuroleptics, given as maintenance treatment, reduce the effect of stressors in producing relapse.
E. There is an association between expressed emotion in a relative and the level of autonomic arousal in the patient.

5.23

A. T – Capgras syndrome was described by Capgras and Reboul-Lachaux in 1923 – they called it *l'illusion des sosies*.
B. T – A review of case studies reports a preponderance of females.
C. F – Delusional memories concern past rather than present events.
D. T – The average age of onset is later than for other schizophrenics.
E. F – If there is evidence of cerebral dysfunction, it is always located in the right hemisphere.

Further reading: Cutting (1990; pp. 214–219)

5.24

A. T – The World Health Organization cross-cultural comparison based on 1400 schizophrenics making a first contact with any treatment agency indicates this.
B. F – Schizophrenia is equally common in men and women.
C. F – Patients with schizophrenia show an excess of births in winter and early spring. This effect is more marked in patients without a family history of the illness.
D. F – There is a negative association.
E. T.

Further reading: Sartorius *et al.* (1986); Kendall (1993; pp. 397–426)

5.25

A. F – The course of the illness seems to be more favourable in less developed countries.
B. F – This applies to first episodes and to relapses.
C. T – And an overstimulating environment can lead to relapse.
D. T – This has been shown for life events and high expressed emotion in relatives.
E. T – This suggests that such arousal may be a mediating factor.

Further reading: World Health Organization (1979); Jablensky *et al.* (1986); Gelder *et al.* (1989; pp. 311–314)

5.26 In schizophrenia, negative symptoms:

A. Include poverty of speech.
B. Include flat affect.
C. Do not respond to antipsychotic treatment.
D. Can be assessed using the SANS.
E. Do not occur in association with positive symptoms.

5.27 The following factors increase the possibility of an unusually prolonged or intense grief reaction:

A. The death is sudden or unexpected.
B. The survivor is well-adjusted and can express feelings easily.
C. The survivor is still coming to terms with another bereavement.
D. Death in hospital.
E. Parent dies leaving children aged between 15 and 20.

5.28 The following conditions are particularly likely to be followed by depression:

A. Influenza.
B. Infectious mononucleosis.
C. Parkinson's disease.
D. Hyperthyroidism.
E. Cushing's syndrome.

5.26

A. T.
B. T – Poverty of speech and flat affect are the two symptoms included in all operationalized definitions of negative symptoms.
C. F – Negative symptoms have been reported to diminish with treatment.
D. T – Negative symptoms can be assessed using the Scale for the Assessment of Negative Symptoms (SANS: Andreasen and Olsen, 1982).
E. F – Both frequently occur in schizophrenia.

Further reading: Andreasen (1982); Andreasen and Olsen (1982); Grossman *et al.* (1989); McGlashen and Fenton (1992)

5.27

A. T.
B. F.
C. T.
D. F – Death in hospital does not increase the possibility of an unusually prolonged or intense grief reaction in itself. However, a painful, horrifying or mismanaged death does.
E. F – An increased risk is seen when a parent (especially mother) dies, leaving children aged between 0 and 5 or 10 and 15.

Further reading: Parkes CM (1985)

5.28

A. T – Depression appears to be common after influenza and may sometimes be refractory to treatment.
B. T.
C. T – This is a well-established association.
D. F – The restlessness, irritability and distractibility of hyperthyroidism may resemble anxiety disorder. Depression occurs occasionally.
E. T – Depression is the most frequent psychiatric symptom and paranoid features are common.

Further reading: Lishman (1987; pp. 303, 437); Gelder *et al.* (1989; pp. 243, 379)

5.29 An excess of life events has been reported before the onset of the following:

A. Depressive disorder.
B. Schizophrenia.
C. A first manic episode.
D. Neurosis.
E. Suicide attempt.

5.30 The following statements are correct:

A. Agitated depression is seen more commonly in younger patients.
B. After recovery from depressive stupor patients are able to recall the events which took place during the period of stupor.
C. Schizoaffective disorders (*ICD-10*) are disorders in which both affective and schizophrenic symptoms are prominent within the same period of illness.
D. Patients suffering from recurrent schizoaffective disorder, manic type, rarely develop a defect state.
E. Anxiety may be a symptom in all degrees of depressive disorder.

5.31 The following statements about depression are correct:

A. Depression is twice as common in women as in men.
B. The prevalence is higher in rural than in urban areas.
C. There is no association between unemployment and depressive symptoms.
D. There is evidence of major differences in symptomatology between cultures.
E. A higher prevalence in working-class than in middle-class women has been reported.

5.29

A. T – An excess of life events has been shown in the months before the onset of depressive disorder, suicide attempts, the onset of neurosis and schizophrenia.
B. T.
C. T – Ambelas (1987) has shown an association between the first manic episode and reported life events. Later episodes precipitated by life events seemed to require smaller amounts of stress.
D. T.
E. T.

Further reading: Ambelas (1987); Gelder *et al.* (1989; pp. 240–243)

5.30

A. F – Seen more commonly among the middle-aged and elderly.
B. T.
C. T.
D. T.
E. T – But can be just as severe in mild depressive disorders as in severe ones.

Further reading: Gelder *et al.* (1989; pp. 221–225, 288–289); World Health Organization (1992)

5.31

A. T – The difference is maximal in young adults and is considerably reduced in old age.
B. F – The prevalence is higher in urban areas, for reasons which are still obscure.
C. F – Unemployment is associated with an increased prevalence of depressive symptoms.
D. F – Although somatic symptoms may dominate the clinical picture in Africa and Asia.
E. T.

Further reading: Kendall (1993; pp. 435–437)

5.32 Borderline personality disorder (*DSM-IV*):

A. Is more commonly diagnosed in women than in men.
B. Is as common in the relatives of schizophrenics as in the treated relatives of borderline patients.
C. Is commonly diagnosed in patients who later go on to develop schizophrenia.
D. Is commonly associated with other personality disorders.
E. Is associated with substance abuse.

5.33 The following are true of phobic anxiety disorders:

A. The individual experiences anticipatory anxiety.
B. Phobic anxiety is indistinguishable from other types of anxiety.
C. The individual avoids circumstances which provoke anxiety.
D. Paranoia is a common symptom.
E. Phobic anxiety is the same as normal fear.

5.32

A. T.
B. F – Borderline personality occurs more commonly in the treated relatives of borderline patients than in the relatives of schizophrenic patients.
C. F – Several studies show that only a minority of borderline patients develop schizophrenia.
D. T – Many people who meet *DSM-IV* criteria for borderline personality disorder also meet criteria for histrionic, narcissistic and antisocial personality disorder.
E. T – Affective features, eating disorders and substance abuse appear to co-occur with borderline personality disorder.

Further reading: Tarnopolsky and Berelowitz (1987); Gelder *et al.* (1989; pp. 137–138); Higgitt and Fonagy (1992)

5.33

A. T – When confronted with the situations which provoke anxiety.
B. T – Phobic anxiety is indistinguishable subjectively and physiologically from other types of anxiety.
C. T.
D. F.
E. F – In phobic anxiety the fear is out of proportion to the situation, cannot be reasoned away and is beyond voluntary control.

Further reading: Gelder *et al.* (1989; pp. 183–184); Freeman (1993; pp. 485–524)

5.34 Characteristic symptoms of panic disorder include:

A. Depersonalization.
B. Feelings of choking.
C. Trembling or shaking.
D. Dizziness.
E. Fear of losing control.

5.35 Obsessive-compulsive disorder:

A. Does not occur more frequently in the families of patients.
B. Occurs more commonly in men than in women.
C. Often has a fluctuating course.
D. Is best treated with clomipramine alone.
E. Occurs more commonly in individuals of lower social class and intelligence.

5.34

A. T.
B. T.
C. T.
D. T.
E. T.

Note: All the above are *DSM-IV* symptoms of panic attack.

Further reading: American Psychiatric Association (1994); World Health Organization (1992); Freeman (1993; pp. 485–524)

5.35

A. F – Obsessive-compulsive disorder occurs slightly more frequently in parents of affected individuals, when compared with the general population.
B. F – The proportions of men and women are roughly equal, but they differ in some obsessive-compulsive subtypes.
C. T.
D. F – Obsessional rituals usually improve with a combination of exposure to any environmental cues and response prevention. Drug effects with clomipramine are modest and occur only in patients with definite depressive symptoms.
E. F – Several studies suggest that individuals with obsessive-compulsive disorder are of above average social class and intelligence.

Further reading: Marks (1987; pp. 424–426); Gelder *et al.* (1989; pp. 196–202); Freeman (1993; pp. 485–525)

5.36 Characteristic features of post-traumatic stress disorder (PTSD) (*ICD-10*) include:

A. Autonomic signs of severe anxiety.
B. Vivid nightmares.
C. Stupor.
D. Onset immediately after the stressful event.
E. Avoidance of reminders of the stressful event.

5.37 Characteristic features of koro include:

A. Delusions that the penis will retract into the abdomen.
B. Echolalia.
C. It occurs mainly at night.
D. Fear of imminent death.
E. Episodes of acute anxiety.

5.36

A. F – This is a feature of an acute stress reaction, which occurs after a major stressful event. Symptoms usually resolve within 2–3 days of the removal of stress.
B. T – Characteristic features include recurrent upsetting dreams and nightmares, intrusive memories and flashbacks of the traumatic events.
C. F – A feature of acute stress reaction.
D. F – A feature of an acute stress reaction. In PTSD the onset is usually delayed, i.e. there is a latency period lasting weeks to months after the stressful event, before the onset of PTSD.
E. T – Also increased arousal, insomnia and depression.

Further reading: World Health Organization (1992); Freeman (1993; pp. 518–519)

5.37

A. F – Koro is a culture-bound syndrome which characteristically occurs in men in South-west Asia, especially the Chinese. It is characterized by episodes of acute anxiety during which the sufferer believes that his penis will retract into his abdomen and cause death. This belief is not a delusion.
B. F – This is seen in latah, which occurs in women in Malaysia. The onset is usually after a frightening experience and features include echolalia and echopraxia.
C. T – Most episodes occur at night.
D. T.
E. T – The patient experiences episodes of acute anxiety which are accompanied by sweating, palpitations, pericardial discomfort and trembling.

Further reading: Gelder *et al.* (1989; pp. 195–196, 208); World Health Organization (1992)

5.38 Dopamine receptor agonists:
A. Include reserpine.
B. Include bromocriptine.
C. Commonly produce vomiting.
D. Stimulate prolactin production.
E. Include orphenadrine.

5.39 Tardive dyskinesia:
A. Is thought to be a consequence of prolonged antipsychotic treatment.
B. Should be treated with antiparkinsonian agents.
C. Can occur in people who have never taken any antipsychotic drug.
D. Is best treated by increasing antipsychotic medication.
E. Is commoner in elderly patients on antipsychotics.

5.38

A. F – Reserpine depletes the brain tissue stores of dopamine, and also of noradrenaline, 5-HT and histamine.
B. T.
C. T – Dopamine receptor agonists commonly produce vomiting. Antagonists such as phenothiazines and metoclopramide are effective antiemetics. It is probable that the medullary dopaminergic pathway is associated with emesis.
D. F – Dopamine receptor agonists stimulate pituitary receptors in the hypothalamic-hypophyseal pathway and inhibit prolactin release.
E. F – This is an anticholinergic agent.

Further reading: Silverstone and Turner (1988; pp. 13, 37, 110–117)

5.39

A. T – Tardive dyskinesia is a disorder involving the extrapyramidal system. Hyperkinetic involuntary movements occur in the oral, facial, buccal and lingual areas and there may also be involuntary movements of the trunk and extremities. It is generally thought to be associated with long-term antipsychotic treatment but has been reported in individuals who have never taken these drugs. The basic mechanism is thought to be hypersensitivity of the dopamine receptors in the nigrostriatal system.
B. F – This only worsens the condition.
C. T.
D. F – This may improve the condition in the short term but has no long-term benefits. The best strategy is to stop the medication and wait for the condition to improve spontaneously.
E. T.

Further reading: Silverstone and Turner (1988; pp. 127–129)

5.40 The following drugs possess antipsychotic properties:
A. Tetrabenazine.
B. Oxypertine.
C. Amitriptyline.
D. Clozapine.
E. Buspirone.

5.41 Acute lithium toxicity typically causes:
A. Seizures.
B. Tardive dyskinesia.
C. Cardiac arrhythmias.
D. Hyperglycaemia.
E. Myxoedema.

5.42 The following drugs can increase lithium levels:
A. Indomethacin.
B. Thiazides.
C. Theophylline.
D. Phenytoin.
E. Chlorpromazine.

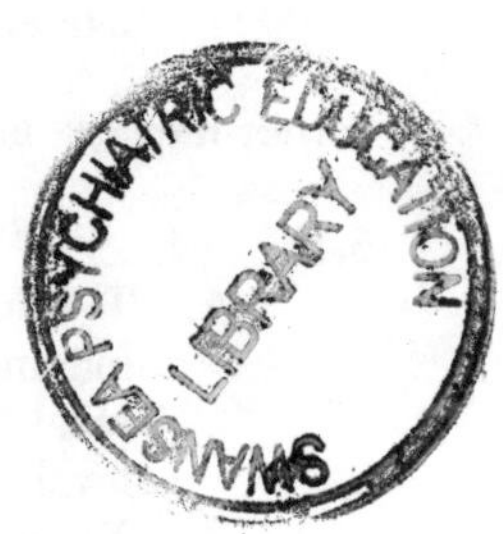

5.40

A. T – This is a synthetic benzoquinolizine which depletes the brain of its monoamine stores.
B. T – This is an indole derivative, which appears to possess antipsychotic properties.
C. F – This is a tricyclic antidepressant.
D. T.
E. F.

Further reading: Silverstone and Turner (1988; pp. 110–117)

5.41

A. T – Acute intoxication is characterized by vomiting, profuse diarrhoea, coarse tremor, ataxia, coma and seizures.
B. F.
C. T.
D. F – This is not a toxic effect. Lithium, if anything, has a weak insulin-like action.
E. F – Although lithium can cause hypothyroidism, this is a late effect.

Further reading: Baldessarini (1990; pp. 420–421)

5.42

A. T – Some non-steroidal anti-inflammatory drugs, e.g. indomethacin and phenylbutazone, can facilitate proximal renal tubular resorption of lithium, thus increasing plasma levels.
B. T – Lithium excretion is reduced by loop diuretics and thiazides, thus causing increased plasma levels and risk of toxicity.
C. F – Lithium excretion is increased with a consequent reduced plasma concentration.
D. F – Neurotoxicity can occur without increased plasma lithium concentration.
E. F.

Further reading: Baldessarini (1990; p. 420); *British National Formulary* (1994; pp. 161–162)

5.43 The following are true of benzodiazepines:

A. Chronic use is associated with reduced hypnotic effect.
B. Chronic use is associated with reduced anticonvulsant effect.
C. Physical dependence has been reported after a treatment period of 1 month.
D. They lead to decreased beta activity on the EEG.
E. Increased time is spent in REM sleep.

5.44 The following statements about benzodiazepines are true:

A. Benzodiazepine receptor proteins are heterogeneous.
B. Benzodiazepine receptors in the CNS are concentrated in the limbic system.
C. Most benzodiazepine receptors are coupled to the GABA receptor and the chloride channel in a GABA/benzodiazepine receptor/chloride channel complex.
D. The GABA/benzodiazepine receptor/chloride channel complex mediates the anxiolytic effects of benzodiazepines.
E. Only pharmacologically active benzodiazepines interact with benzodiazepine receptors.

5.45 The following drugs can react with tricyclic antidepressants:

A. Oral contraceptives.
B. Phenytoin.
C. Propranolol.
D. Disulfiram.
E. Metformin.

5.43

A. T.
B. T.
C. T.
D. F – Benzodiazepines cause a decrease in alpha activity and an increase in beta activity.
E. F – This time is decreased.

Further reading: Silverstone and Turner (1988; pp. 190–191); Rall (1990; p. 349)

5.44

A. T.
B. F – All brain structures investigated appear to have some benzodiazepine receptors in varying numbers.
C. T.
D. T – This complex can also mediate anxiety.
E. F – Benzodiazepine receptor antagonists also interact with the receptors.

Further reading: Braestrup and Nielsen (1982)

5.45

A. T – Oral contraceptives antagonize the antidepressant effect of tricyclics.
B. T – Phenytoin reduces plasma concentrations of tricyclics. Tricyclics antagonize the anticonvulsant action of phenytoin (by lowering the seizure threshold).
C. F – But plasma concentrations of propanolol are increased by fluvoxamine (serotonin re-uptake inhibitor).
D. T – Disulfiram inhibits the metabolism of tricyclics.
E. F – MAOIs enhance the hypoglycaemic effect

Further reading: *British National Formulary* (1994; pp. 507–508)

5.46 The following are midbrain structures:
A. Corpora quadrigemina.
B. Nucleus dentatus.
C. Oculomotor nuclear complex.
D. Inferior olivary nucleus.
E. Red nucleus.

5.47 Efferent components of the direct and consensual light reflex include:
A. Oculomotor nerve fibres.
B. Ciliary ganglion.
C. Optic nerve fibres.
D. Superior colliculus.
E. Lateral geniculate body.

5.46

A. T – These are four rounded elevations, the paired superior and inferior colliculi, which are located on the dorsal surface of the midbrain.
B. F – The dentate nucleus is situated in the cerebellum.
C. T – The nucleus of the oculomotor nerve is situated in the midbrain, anterior to the grey matter, in the region of the superior colliculus.
D. F – The inferior olivary nucleus is situated in the medulla.
E. T – The red nucleus is a prominent motor component of the tegmentum. It is egg-shaped and extends from the caudal limit of the superior colliculus into the subthalamic region of the diencephalon.

Further reading: Barr and Kiernan (1988; pp. 90, 96, 113, 122–123, 167)

5.47

A. T – Efferent impulses travel in fibres of the oculomotor nerve to the ciliary ganglion. From there the postganglionic fibres reach the sphincter pupillae muscle of the iris, causing constriction of the pupil.
B. T.
C. F – Afferent impulses travel in the optic nerve to visceral oculomotor neurones on both sides.
D. F.
E. F.

Further reading: Brodal (1981; pp. 560–564); Barr and Kiernan (1988; pp. 128–129)

5.48 Cerebellar lesions typically cause:

A. Impaired ipsilateral coordination.
B. Resting tremor.
C. Truncal ataxia.
D. Scanning speech.
E. Peripheral neuropathy.

5.49 Characteristic neuropathological features of idiopathic Parkinson's disease include:

A. Cellular degeneration of the substantia nigra.
B. Narrowing of the corpus callosum.
C. Presence of Lewy hyaline inclusion bodies.
D. Neurofibrillary changes.
E. The brain is of normal size.

5.50 Characteristic neuropathological features of Wilson's disease include:

A. Neuronal loss in the caudate and putamen.
B. The brain looks shrunken.
C. Neurofibrillary tangles.
D. The presence of Alzheimer's nuclei.
E. Pericapillary concretions staining for iron.

5.48

A. T.
B. F – Intention tremor is produced and is elicited by the finger–nose and heel–shin tests. Resting tremor occurs in Parkinson's disease. It is present when the patient is sitting quietly and increases when the patient makes voluntary movements.
C. T.
D. T – This can be distinguished from dysarthria, found in bulbar and pseudobulbar palsies.
E. F – Peripheral neuropathy is not a sign of a cerebellar syndrome but can occur in conjunction with ataxia, nystagmus and memory impairment in the Wernicke–Korsakoff syndrome.

Further reading: Barr and Kiernan (1988; pp. 176–177)

5.49

A. T.
B. F – Seen in Huntington's chorea.
C. T.
D. F – Seen in postencephalitic Parkinson's disease.
E. F – Diffuse cortical atrophy is common.

Further reading: Lishman (1987; p. 552)

5.50

A. T – Microscopically there is neuronal loss in the caudate and putamen. Astrocytic nuclei, with a vesicular appearance (Alzheimer nuclei) are seen in the putamen.
B. F – Externally the brain usually looks normal.
C. F.
D. T.
E. F – Pericapillary concretions staining for copper and large phagocytic cells (Opalski cells) are also seen.

Note: In the substantia nigra, phagocytes containing iron pigment are seen. Foci of degeneration are seen in the frontal lobes.

Further reading: Lishman (1987; pp. 563–567)

References

Ackner, B. (1954) Depersonalization: I aetiology and phenomenology. *Journal of Mental Science* **100**, 838–872. [3.1]

Adams, R.D & Victor, M. (1989) *Principles of Neurology*, 4th edn. New York: McGraw-Hill. [1.6: 1.17: 1.18: 2.3: 3.3]

Addonizio, G., Susman, V.L. & Roth, S.D. (1987) Neuroleptic malignant syndrome: review and analysis of 115 cases. *Biological Psychiatry* **22**, 1004–1020. [1.24]

Ambelas, A.C. (1987) Life events and mania. A special relationship? *British Journal of Psychiatry* **150**, 235–240. [5.29]

American Psychiatric Association (1994) *Diagnostic and Statistical Manual of Mental Disorders*, 4th edn (*DSM-IV*). Washington, DC: APA. [1.31: 2.32: 2.37: 3.32: 4.32: 5.22: 5.34]

Andreasen, N.C. (1979a) Thought, language and communication disorders. I. Clinical assessment, definition of terms and evaluation of their reliability. *Archives of General Psychiatry* **36**, 1315–1321. [3.24]

Andreasen, N.C. (1979b) Thought, language and communication disorders II. Diagnostic significance. *Archives of General Psychiatry* **36**, 1325–1330. [3.24]

Andreasen, N.C. (1982) Negative symptoms in schizophrenia. *Archives of General Psychiatry* **39**, 784–788. [5.26]

Andreasen, N.C. & Olsen, S. (1982) Negative versus positive schizophrenia: definition and validation. *Archives of General Psychiatry* **39**, 789–794. [5.26]

Baldessarini, R.J. (1990) Drugs and the treatment of psychiatric disorders. In: *Goodman and Gilman's The Pharmacological Basis of Therapeutics*, 8th edn (Goodman Gilman, A., Rall, T.W., Nies, A.S. & Taylor, P., eds), pp. 383–435. New York: Pergamon Press. [1.41: 1.42: 2.40: 2.41: 2.42: 3.40: 3.42: 3.44: 4.40: 4.41: 4.42: 5.41: 5.42]

Baldwin, R.C. (1991) Affective disorders: depressive illness. In: *Psychiatry in the Elderly* (Jacoby, R. & Oppenheimer, C., eds), pp. 676–719. Oxford: Oxford University Press. [3.31]

Barnes, T.R.E. & Braude, W.M. (1985) Akathisia variants and tardive dyskinesia. *Archives of General Psychiatry* **42**, 874–878. [2.22]

Barr, M.L. & Kiernan, J.A. (1988) *The Human Nervous System. An Anatomical Viewpoint*, 5th edn. Philadelphia, PA: J.B. Lippincott. [1.46: 1.47: 2.45: 2.46: 2.47: 3.46: 3.48: 4.46: 4.47: 4.48: 5.46: 5.47: 5.48]

Beck, A.T. (1967) *Depression: Clinical, Experimental and Theoretical Aspects*. New York: Hoeber Medical Division (Harper & Row). [1.27]

Berlyne, N. (1972) Confabulation. *British Journal of Psychiatry* **120**, 31–39. [1.6]

Bertelsen, A., Harvald, B. & Hauge, M. (1977) A Danish twin study of manic-depressive disorders. *British Journal of Psychiatry* **136**, 330–351. [4.27]

Braestrup, C. & Nielsen, M. (1982) Anxiety. *Lancet* **ii**, 1030–1034. [5.44]

British National Formulary (1994) Number 28. London: British Medical Association and the Royal Pharmaceutical Society of Great Britain. [1.41: 1.43: 2.39: 2.41: 2.44: 4.39: 4.40: 4.45: 5.42: 5.45]

Brockington, I. (1986) Diagnosis of schizophrenia and schizoaffective psychoses. In: *The Psychopharmacology and Treatment of Schizophrenia* (Bradley, P.B. & Hirsch, S.R., eds), pp. 166–199. Oxford: Oxford University Press. [4.21]

Brodal, A. (1981) *Neurological Anatomy in Relation to Clinical Medicine*, 3rd edn. New York: Oxford University Press. [1.47: 2.45: 3.46: 3.47: 4.48: 5.47]

Brown, J.A.C. (1961) *Freud and the post-Freudians.* Harmondsworth: Penguin Books. [1.14]

Brown, D. & Pedder, J. (1991) *Introduction to Psychotherapy*, 2nd edn. London: Routledge. [1.9: 1.10: 1.11: 1.12: 2.9: 2.11: 2.12: 3.9: 3.10: 3.11: 3.12: 3.13: 4.9: 4.10: 4.11: 5.10: 5.11: 5.12: 5.13: 5.14]

Campbell, I.C. & Reveley, M.A. (1984) Neuropharmacology. In: *The Scientific Principles of Psychopathology* (McGuffin, P., Shanks, M.F. & Hodgson, R.J., eds), pp. 97–136. London: Grune & Stratton. [3.41]

Clare, A. (1993) Interpretative psychotherapies. In: *Companion to Psychiatric Studies*, 5th edn (Kendall R.E. & Zealley, A.K., eds), pp. 879–898. Edinburgh: Churchill Livingstone. [1.13]

Coger, R.W. & Serafetinides, E.A. (1990) Schizophrenia, corpus callosum, and interhemispheric communication: a review. *Psychiatry Research* **34**, 163–184. [1.21]

Cox, J.L. (1993) Psychiatric disorders of childbirth. In: *Companion to Psychiatric Studies*, 5th edn (Kendall, R.E. & Zealley, A.K., eds), pp. 577–586. Edinburgh: Churchill Livingstone. [3.30]

Cutting, J. (1987) The phenomenology of acute organic psychosis. *British Journal of Psychiatry* **151**, 324–332. [5.6]

Cutting, J. (1989) Hearing voices (editorial). *British Medical Journal* **298**, 769–770. [4.1: 5.1]

Cutting, J. (1990) *The Right Cerebral Hemisphere and Psychiatric Disorders.* Oxford: Oxford University Press. [5.23]

Davison, K. & Bagley, C.R. (1969) Schizophrenia-like psychoses associated with organic disorders of the central nervous system: a review of the literature. In: *Current Problems in Neuropsychiatry* (Herrington, R.N., ed.). British Journal of Psychiatry special publication no. 4, pp. 113–184. Ashford, Kent: Headley Brothers. [5.15]

Dean, C. & Kendall, R.E. (1981) The symptomatology of puerperal illnesses. *British Journal of Psychiatry* **139**, 128–133. [1.28]

de Mare, P. (1984) Large group perspectives. In: *Spheres of Group Analysis* (Lear, T.E., ed.), pp. 45–49. Naas, Kildare: Group Analytic Society Publications. [2.13]

Duchen, L.W. & Jacobs, J.M. (1992) Nutritional deficiencies and metabolic disorders. In: *Greenfield's Neuropathology*, 5th edn (Hume Adams, J. & Duchen, L.W., eds), pp. 811–880. London: Edward Arnold. [1.49: 2.49]

Easton, M.S. (1990) Seasonal affective disorders. *Current Opinion in Psychiatry* **3**, 54–57. [1.29]

Elphick, M. (1989) Clinical issues in the use of carbamazepine in psychiatry: a review. *Psychological Medicine* **19**, 591–604. [2.43]

Endicott, J. & Spitzer, R.L. (1978) A diagnostic interview: the schedule for affective disorders and schizophrenia. *Archives of General Psychiatry* **35**, 837–844. [5.21: 5.22]

Enoch, M.D. & Trethowan, W. (1991) *Uncommon Psychiatric Syndromes*, 3rd edn. Oxford: Butterworth-Heinemann. [1.36: 2.4: 2.30]

Esiri, M.M. & Kennedy, P.G.E. (1992) Virus diseases. In: *Greenfield's Neuropathology*, 5th edn (Hume Adams, J. & Duchen, L.E., eds), pp. 335–399. London: Edward Arnold. [3.49]

Feighner, J.P., Robins, E., Guze, S.B., Woodruff, R.A., Winokur, G. & Munoz, R. (1972) Diagnostic criteria for use in psychiatric research. *Archives of General Psychiatry* **26**, 57–63. [5.21: 5.22]

Fenton, G.W. (1993) Epilepsy and psychiatric disorder. In: *Companion to Psychiatric Studies*, 5th edn (Kendall, R.E. & Zealley, A.K., eds), pp. 343–358. Edinburgh: Churchill Livingstone. [3.6: 5.5]

File, S. (1988) The benzodiazepine receptor and its role in anxiety. *British Journal of Psychiatry* **152**, 599–600. [1.45]

Fish, F. (1984) *Outline of Psychiatry for Students and Practitioners*, 4th edn. (Hamilton, M., ed.) Bristol: Wright

Fish, F. (1985) *Clinical Psychopathology: Signs and Symptoms in Psychiatry*, 2nd edn. (Hamilton, M., ed.). Bristol: Wright

Freeman, C.P.L. (1993) Neurotic disorders. In: *Companion to Psychiatric Studies*, 5th edn (Kendall, R.E. & Zealley, A.K., eds), pp. 485–524. Edinburgh: Churchill Livingstone. [1.33: 1.35: 1.37: 2.34: 2.35: 2.36: 2.37: 3.36: 3.38: 4.36: 5.33: 5.34: 5.35: 5.36]

Gelder, M., Gath, D. & Mayou, R. (1989) *Oxford Textbook of Psychiatry*, 2nd edn. Oxford: Oxford University Press. [1.2: 1.7: 1.10: 1.19: 1.20: 1.21: 1.22: 1.24: 1.26: 1.27: 1.29: 1.30: 1.33: 1.34: 1.35: 1.37: 2.2: 2.6: 2.16: 2.18: 2.19: 2.20: 2.21: 2.25: 2.27: 2.28: 2.29: 2.34: 2.35: 2.36: 2.37: 3.2: 3.15: 3.16: 3.19: 3.20: 3.21: 3.22: 3.25: 3.27: 3.33: 3.34: 3.35: 3.36: 3.38: 4.2: 4.5: 4.7: 4.8: 4.20: 4.21: 4.31: 4.34: 4.35: 4.36: 4.37: 5.4: 5.6: 5.7: 5.25: 5.28: 5.29: 5.30: 5.32: 5.33: 5.35: 5.37]

Gibb, W.R.G. (1988) Neuroleptic malignant syndrome in striatonignal degeneration . *British Journal of Psychiatry* **153**, 254–255. [1.24]

Gilman, S. & Winans, S. (1982) *Manter & Gatz's Essentials of Clinical Neuroanatomy and Neurophysiology*, 6th edn. Philadelphia, PA: F.A. Davis. [1.48]

Glass, I.B. (1989a) Alcoholic hallucinosis: a psychiatric enigma. 1. The development of the idea. *British Journal of Addiction* **84**, 29–41. [2.8]

Glass, I.B. (1989b) Alcoholic hallucinosis: a psychiatric enigma. 2. Follow up studies. *British Journal of Addiction* **84**, 151–164. [2.8]

Glass, I.B. & Marshall, E.J. (1991) Alcohol and mental illness: cause or effect? In: *The International Handbook of Addictive Behaviour* (Glass, I.B., ed.), pp. 152–162. London: Routledge. [2.8]

Grossman, L.S., Luchins, D.J. & Harrow, M. (1989) Positive and negative symptoms and the neurology and schizophrenia. *Current Opinion in Psychiatry* **2**, 20–25. [5.26]

Gunnell, D., Frankel, S. (1994) Presentation of suicide: aspirations and evidence. *British Medical Journal* **308**, 1227–1233 [4.31]

Hanson, D. (1988) Causes and consequences of late onset involuntary motor movements in schizophrenic patients. *Current Opinion in Psychiatry* **1**, 32–40. [2.22]

Hawton, K. (1992) By their own young hand. *British Medical Journal* **304**, 1000 [4.31]

Hay, G.G. (1970) Dysmorphophobia. *British Journal of Psychiatry* **116**, 399–406. [4.7]

Higgitt, A. & Fonagy, P. (1992) Psychotherapy in borderline and narcissistic personality disorder. *British Journal of Psychiatry* **161**, 23–43. [5.32]

House, A. (1987) Depression after stroke. *British Medical Journal* **294**, 76–78. [3.29]

House, A., Dennis, M., Mogridge, L. *et al.* (1991) Mood disorders in the first year after stroke. *British Journal of Psychiatry* **158**, 83–92

Insel, T.R. & Akiskal, H.S. (1986) Obsessive-compulsive disorder with psychotic features: a phenomenologic analysis. *American Journal of Psychiatry* **143**, 1527–1533. [1.32]

Jablensky, A., Korten, A., Ernberg, G. *et al.* (1986) Manifestations and first-contact incidence of schizophrenia in different cultures. *Psychological Medicine* **16**, 909–928. [5.25]

Keck, P.E., Pope, H.G., Cohen, B.M. *et al.* (1989) Risk factors for neuroleptic malignant syndrome. *Archives of General Psychiatry* **46**, 914–918. [1.24]

Kendall, R.E. (1993) Mood (affective) disorders. In: *Companion to Psychiatric Studies*, 5th edn (Kendall, R.E. & Zealley, A.K., eds), pp. 427–458. Edinburgh: Churchill Livingstone. [5.31]

Kendall, R.E. (1993) Schizophrenia. In: *Companion to Psychiatric Studies*, 5th edn (Kendall, R.E. & Zealley, A.K., eds), pp. 397–426. Edinburgh: Churchill Livingstone. [1.23: 2.24: 3.23: 3.24: 4.23: 4.24: 5.22: 5.24]

Kräupl-Taylor, F. (1979) *Psychopathology. Its Causes and Symptoms* (revised edn). Middlesex, England: Quartermaine House. [3.3: 3.5: 4.4: 5.3]

Kräupl-Taylor, F. (1981) On pseudohallucinations. *Psychological Medicine* **11**, 265–271. [1.8]

Kräupl-Taylor, F. (1983) Descriptive and developmental phenomena. In: *Handbook of Psychiatry, Volume I. General Psychopathology* (Shepherd, M & Zangwill, O.L., eds), pp. 59–94. Cambridge: Cambridge University Press. [4.3: 5.8]

Krauthammer, C. & Klerman, G.L. (1978) Secondary mania. *Archives of General Psychiatry* **35**, 1333–1339. [3.28: 4.28]

Lader, M. (1987) Clinical pharmacology of benzodiazepines. *Annual Reviews in Medicine* **38**, 19–28. [3.45]

Lahmeyer, H.W. & Lilie, J.K. (1991) Seasonal affective disorders. *Current Opinion in Psychiatry* **4**, 56–59. [4.29]

Liebowitz, M.R., Gorman, J.M., Fyer, A.J. & Klein, O.F. (1985) Social phobia. *Archives of General Psychiatry* **42**, 729–736. [2.35]

Lishman, W.A. (1987) *Organic Psychiatry*, 2nd edn. Oxford: Blackwell. [1.6: 1.15: 1.16: 1.17: 1.18: 1.36: 1.49: 1.50: 2.5: 2.6: 2.15: 2.16: 2.17: 2.18: 2.48: 2.49: 2.50: 3.4: 3.7: 3.8: 3.17: 3.18: 3.19: 3.29: 3.37: 3.49: 3.50: 4.5: 4.6: 4.8: 4.15: 4.16: 4.17: 4.18: 4.19: 4.49: 4.50: 5.4: 5.5: 5.15: 5.16: 5.17: 5.18: 5.19: 5.20: 5.28: 5.49: 5.50]

McDougle, C.J. & Goodman, W.K. (1990) Obsessive-compulsive disorder: recent neurobiological developments. *Current Opinion in Psychiatry* **3**, 239–244. {1.32]

McDougle, C.J. & Goodman, W.K. (1991) Obsessive compulsive disorders: pharmacotherapy and pathophysiology. *Current Opinion in Psychiatry* **4**, 267–272. [1.32]

McGlashan, T.H. & Fenton, W.S. (1992) The positive–negative distinction in schizophrenia. *Archives of General Psychiatry* **49**, 63–72. [2.23: 5.26]

McKenna, P.J. (1984) Disorders with overvalued ideas. *British Journal of Psychiatry* **145**, 579–585. [2.7: 4.7: 5.7]

Mann, S.C., Caroff, S.N., Bleier, H.R. *et al.* (1986) Lethal catatonia. *American Journal of Psychiatry* **143**, 1374–1381. [1.24]

Manschreck, T.C., Maher, B.A., Rucklos, M.E. & Vereen, D.R. (1982) Disturbed voluntary motor activity in schizophrenic disorder. *Psychological Medicine* **12**, 73–84. [2.25]

Marks, I.M. (1987) *Fears, Phobias and Rituals: Panic, Anxiety and their Disorders.* New York: Oxford University Press. [1.35: 2.36: 3.36: 4.36: 5.35]

Martin, J.B. (1984) Huntington's disease: new approaches to an old problem. *Neurology* **34**, 1059–1072. [1.16: 2.16]

Meats, P. (1988) Olfactory hallucinations (letter). *British Medical Journal* **296**, 645. [1.1]

Mellor, C.S. (1970) First rank symptoms of schizophrenia. *British Journal of Psychiatry* **117**, 15–23. [4.23]

Mellor, C.S. (1982) The present status of first rank symptoms. *British Journal of Psychiatry* **140**, 423–424. [4.23]

Morgan, H.G. (1983) General medical disorders. In: *Handbook of Psychiatry, Volume 2. Mental Disorders and Somatic Illness* (Lader, M.H., ed.), pp. 14–36. Cambridge: Cambridge University Press. [4.37]

Morice, R.D. & Ingram, J.C.L. (1982) Language analysis in schizophrenia: diagnostic implications. *Australian and New Zealand Journal of Psychiatry* **16**, 11–21. [3.24:

4.24]
Murray, R.M. & McGuffin, P. (1988) Genetic aspects of psychiatric disorders. In: *Companion to Psychiatric Studies*, 5th edn (Kendall, R.E. & Zealley, A.K., eds), pp. 227–262. Edinburgh: Churchill Livingstone. [4.27]

Naguib, M. & Levy, R. (1991) Paranoid states in the elderly and late paraphrenia. In: *Psychiatry in the Elderly* (Jacoby, R. and Oppenheimer, C., eds), pp. 758–778. Oxford: Oxford University Press. [4.25]

Oppenheimer, D.R. & Esiri, M.M. (1992) Diseases of the basal ganglia, cerebellum and motor neurons. In: *Greenfield's Neuropathology*, 5th edn. (Hume Adams, J. & Duchen, L.W., eds), pp. 988–1045. London: Edward Arnold. [1.50]

Parkes, C.M. (1985) Bereavement. *British Journal of Psychiatry* **146**, 11–17. [1.25: 1.26: 3.26: 4.26: 5.27]

Parkes, J.D. (1985) *Sleep and its Disorders*. London: WB Saunders. [3.19]

Platz, C. & Kendall, R.E. (1988) A matched control follow-up and family study of puerperal psychoses. *British Journal of Psychiatry* **153**, 90–94. [1.28]

Protheroe, C. (1969) Puerperal psychoses: a long term study, 1927–1961. *British Journal of Psychiatry* **115**, 9–30. [1.28]

Pryse-Phillips, W. (1971) An olfactory reference syndrome. *Acta Psychiatrica Scandinavica* **47**, 484–509. [1.1]

Rall, T.W. (1990) Hypnotics and sedatives. In: *Goodman and Gilman's The Pharmacological Basis of Therapeutics*, 8th edn (Goodman Gilman, A., Rall , T.W., Nies, A.S. and Taylor, P., eds), pp. 345–381. New York: Pergamon Press. [4.43: 5.43]

Reid, H. & Fallon, R.J. (1992) Bacterial infections. In: *Greenfield's Neuropathology*, 5th edn (Hume Adams, J. & Duchen, L.W., eds), pp. 302–334. London: Edward Arnold. [3.50]

Reveley, M.A. & Campbell, I.C. (1984) Neurochemistry. In: *The Scientific Principles of Psychopathology* (McGuffin, P., Shanks, M.F. & Hodgson, R.J., eds), pp. 57–95. London: Grune & Stratton. [1.38: 3.39: 4.38]

Roberts, A.H. (1969) *Brain Damage in Boxers*. London: Pitman. [4.15]

Rosenthal, N.E., Sack, D.A., Gillin, J.C. *et al.* (1984) Seasonal affective disorder. *Archives of General Psychiatry* **41**, 72–80. [1.29]

Roy, A. (1979) Hysterical seizures. *Archives of Neurology* **36**, 447–448. [3.37]

Sandler, J., Dare, C. & Holder, A. (1970a) Basic psychoanalytic concepts: I. The extension of clinical concepts outside the psychoanalytic situation. *British Journal of Psychiatry* **116**, 551–554. [5.9]

Sandler, J., Holder, A. & Dare, C. (1970b) Basic psychoanalytic concepts: II. The treatment alliance. *British Journal of Psychiatry* **116**, 555–558. [2.10]

Sandler, J., Holder, A & Dare, C. (1970c) Basic psychoanalytic concepts: III. Transference. *British Journal of Psychiatry* **116**, 667–672. [2.11]

Sandler, J., Holder, A. & Dare, C. (1970d) Basic psychoanalytic concepts: IV. Countertransference. *British Journal of Psychiatry* **117**, 83–88. [3.13]

Sandler, J., Holder, A. & Dare, C. (1970e) Basic psychoanalytic concepts: V. Resistance. *British Journal of Psychiatry* **117**, 215–221. [2.14]

Sandler, J., Holder, A. & Dare, C. (1970f) Basic psychoanalytic concepts: VI. Acting out. *British Journal of Psychiatry* **117**, 329–334. [3.14]

Sandler, J., Holder, A. & Dare, C. (1970g) Basic psychoanalytic concepts: VII. The negative therapeutic reaction. *British Journal of Psychiatry* **117**, 431–435. [4.13]

Sartorius, N., Jablensky, A., Korten, A. *et al.* (1986) Early manifestations and first-contact incidence of schizophrenia in different cultures. *Psychological Medicine* **16**, 909–928. [5.24]

Scott, J. (1988) Chronic depression. *British Journal of Psychiatry* **153**, 287–297. [4.30]

Scott, J., Cole, A. & Eccleston, A. (1991) Dealing with persisting abnormalities of mood. *International Review of Psychiatry* **3**, 19–33. [4.30]

Schneider, K. (1959) *Clinical Psychopathology*. Translated by Hamilton, M.W. New York: Grune & Stratton. [1.3: 4.2: 4.23: 5.2]

Sedman, G. (1970) Theories of depersonalisation: a re-appraisal. *British Journal of Psychiatry* **117**, 1–13. [2.1: 3.1]

Shanks, M.F. (1984) An introduction to the functional morphology of the nervous system. In: *The Scientific Principles of Psychopathology* (McGuffin, P., Shanks, M.F. & Hodgson, R.J., eds), pp. 3–36. London: Grune & Stratton. [2.38]

Silverstone, T. & Turner, P. (1988) *Drug Treatment in Psychiatry*, 4th edn. London: Routledge. [1.38: 1.39: 1.40: 1.44: 2.38: 2.39: 2.40: 2.43: 3.39: 3.41: 3.43: 4.38: 4.44: 4.45: 5.38: 5.39: 5.40: 5.43]

Sims, A. (1988) *Symptoms in the Mind*. London: Baillière Tindall. [1.1: 1.2: 1.3: 1.4: 1.5: 1.6: 1.8: 1.19: 1.20: 2.4: 2.5: 2.7: 2.25: 3.2: 3.7: 5.2: 5.3]

Spitzer, R.L., Endicott, J. & Robins, E. (1978) Research diagnostic criteria: rationale and reliability. *Archives of General Psychiatry* **35**, 773–782. [5.21: 5.22]

Stein, G. (1982) The maternity blues. In: *Motherhood and Mental Illness* (Brockington, I.F. & Kumar, R., eds), pp. 119–154. London: Academic Press. [2.31]

Storr, A. (1979) *The Art of Psychotherapy*. London: Secker & Warburg. [4.14]

Tamminga, C.A. & Thaker, G.K. (1989) Tardive dyskinesia. *Current Opinion in Psychiatry* **2**, 12–16. [4.22]

Tarnopolsky, A. & Berelowitz, M. (1987) Borderline personality. A review of recent research. *British Journal of Psychiatry* **151**, 724–734. [5.32]

Tomlinson, B.E. (1992) Ageing and the dementias. In: *Greenfield's Neuropathology*, 5th edn (Hume Adams, J. & Duchen, L.W., eds), pp. 1284–1410. London: Edward Arnold. [2.48: 2.50: 4.49: 4.50]

Treasure, J. (1992) Anorexia nervosa and bulimia nervosa. *Current Opinion in Psychiatry* **5**, 228–233. [4.33]

Tyrer, P. & Murphy, S. (1987) The place of benzodiazepines in psychiatric practice. *British Journal of Psychiatry* **151**, 719–723. [4.43]

Weller, M. (1992) Depressive illness and antidepressant drugs. In: *The Scientific Basis of Psychiatry*, 2nd edn. (Weller, M. & Eysenck, M., eds), pp. 529–557. London: W.B. Saunders. [2.29]

Wigider, T.A., Frances, A.J. & Sweeney, M. (1988) Schizophrenia spectrum disorders. *Current Opinion in Psychiatry* **1**, 13–18. [2.33]

Wing, J.K., Cooper, J.E. & Sartorius, N. (1974) *Measurement and Classification of Psychiatric Symptoms*. Cambridge: Cambridge University Press. [5.22]

World Health Organization (1992) *Schizophrenia: An Initial Follow-up*. Chichester: Wiley. [5.25:]

World Health Organization (1992) *The ICD-10 Classification of Mental and Behavioural Disorders*. Geneva: World Health Organization. [1.7: 1.32: 1.33: 2.4: 2.26: 2.32: 2.34: 2.37: 4.33: 5.25: 5.30: 5.34: 5.36: 5.37]

Yalom, I.D. (1985) *The Theory and Practice of Group Psychotherapy*, 3rd edn. New York: Basic Books. [1.12: 4.12]

Subject index

Note: Question numbers are given instead of page numbers